SEEING THE GOOD IN IT

OASIS BOOKS

An imprint of Oasis Family Media, LLC.

oasisfamilymedia.com

First published in the United States of America by Oasis Books,
an imprint of Oasis Family Media, LLC., 2024

Printed in the United States of America

First printing; June 2024

ISBN: 978-1-63108-634-2

Cover and interior design by Seth Guge

Also available as an audiobook from Oasis Audio wherever audiobooks are sold.

SEEING THE GOOD IN IT

PHIL ZIELKE

OASIS
BOOKS

289 S Main Pl, Carol Stream, IL 60188

Dear Ruth, I dedicate this book in loving memory of you.

You were the adopted grandmother God strategically placed in my neighborhood for me to learn from and grow with. There was so much power in your words. The stories you told always captivated me. Thank you for sharing your challenges and how God brought you through each one in the most unexpected ways. Your father was an expert builder, but so were you—you built into me the idea that there is much purpose to be found in life, even in difficult times. You helped me see where a solid foundation comes from. When I think of you, I can't help but see the good in it.

CONTENTS

INTRODUCTION

I am a firm believer that God can and does use any and all types of situations to accomplish his purpose. I've always been more trusting than not. But when you find out that someone in your family has cancer it certainly does cause one to think. *What? Why? When? How long?* All the usual questions come to mind. We knew there was a problem. We knew that there was a reality. We didn't know what it might be. Phil will tell you that cancer was the best thing that ever happened to him. But for me, a parent, finding out that my son was ill was the beginning of a roller coaster ride. For me, roller coaster rides are ok, but I tend to like to be more in control, not just a passenger on a ride. I don't know how people handle the news of a terminal illness without the message of salvation or the knowledge of God's grace.

I rushed home at the end of one school day to find my son lying in his bed, not feeling well. I flat out told him, "Phil, the doctor called me and told me you have cancer." His reaction was as if he had just heard a joke. "Are you sure? Are you telling me the truth? You're lying, aren't you?" "No, Phil, I wouldn't lie about something like this." His face turned. I asked him to pray with me. We prayed. It was a bit longer than this, but here is what I prayed: "God, we don't know what is in store for us. We got some bad news today. We don't know what your plan is. Please be with Philip and each of us because we need you. Lord, whatever comes of this, help each of us to be a witness for you through it all. Help us sort it out. Give us the strength we need to endure and do what you see best."

How do you find hope when the news you face is one of despair? I

1

think it has something to do with trust. When I was told on the phone by the doctor that the results of the biopsy were conclusive—it was cancer—immediately things began to be set in motion. The Jewish doctor at the University of Chicago Hospital told me to set an appointment with his staff. I tried, but was told that nothing was available. He then called me to inquire why I hadn't just come down to the hospital. He said that he is the one who runs the department and that he would get us in. There are so many things that I can share where it is clearly evident that God is directing the process.

The coaster ride continued with doctor visits. I have never liked to talk with doctors. I have a bit of a hospital phobia. When I would visit someone in the hospital, I would always check to make sure I knew where the exits were just in case I needed to make a quick escape. Going to a doctor raises my blood pressure. But staying overnight in the hospital became a way of life for me. Amazingly I only fainted once during Phil's cancer journey. Somehow I didn't even feel queasy during the first bone marrow test I saw them do on my son. It is kind of amazing the things that I did that were totally contrary to my impulses when the health concerns of my son took on a major heightened role.

Cancer affects the whole family. Priorities change. Phil's health plan changed the way we would live for a couple of years. Looking back, I treasure the witness of those whom I spoke with while waiting at the hospital for Phil to finish a test or get results. I especially remember a man who was an aging organist at his church on the south side of Chicago. He told me about his heart transplant, the complications that went with it, his colon cancer, and his faith. Despite all his difficulties, he talked about the strength he had and how his faith in God got him through.

It is amazing for me to this day, that I never felt that Phil's earthly life was ever in jeopardy. It's strange to say, but I had somewhat of a sense of peace about this whole cancer thing. Even though there were so many unknowns and sometimes life became a fog, I too look back and see Phil's cancer as a growth opportunity for me. Phil certainly had his ups and downs—the moods caused by the poisonous chemicals pumped into his body changed him from day to day. But even with the over-the-speed-limit trips to the hospital, the challenging unknown of medicine reactions, and the stress of juggling work and family, our faith sure did grow.

Is having a life-threatening illness any different than the situation we live with every day of our lives? We are all stuck in the illness of sin from birth as human beings. Yet some of us, those who proclaim Christ, are not stuck, are we? We are set free from the penalty of eternal death that our sin-sick souls deserve. That is why we do what we do. That is why we serve God. We have a purpose in reaching others for Christ.

Where is the hope for people who don't know Christ? How do they survive through the ups and downs and the despairs of life? I can't imagine going through what we did without knowing our Savior. May Phil's story encourage you with the Savior who remained with him every step of the way.

Steve Zielke

CHAPTER 1

MY STORY

For the first part of my life, I was innocent and naive enough to think I was untouchable and invincible. Disease, sickness, setbacks, or afflictions—nothing could possibly slow me down. Nobody could tell me what I couldn't do, and on the rare occasion that someone did, my mission in life was to prove them wrong. When someone told me I couldn't be the best in a high-stakes running competition, I'd run faster; when someone told me I couldn't dunk a basketball, I'd jump higher; when someone told me I couldn't date a certain special girl, I'd find a way. If someone told me I couldn't accomplish a task, it was as if they had lit a match and thrown it onto a pile of dry leaves. It would start out as an inconspicuous spark, but eventually, the entire forest was ablaze. My confidence in myself and my abilities grew just as quickly as that fire. But, being young and naive, I thought my determination, passion, and persistence were enough. How little I understood about life and myself at that time.

I remember setting the bar high for achievement, even as a young child. At the age of eight, I made it my goal to get a scholarship so I could afford college. My dad was a teacher and athletic director in a private school. My mom raised my younger brother, two sisters, and me while working part-time as an aerobics instructor at the local YMCA. My parents' income was low enough that we qualified for government assistance. So, I took it upon myself to pay for my own college education. Through sweat, tears, and sacrifice, I achieved the dream of a college athletic scholarship in track and field. Then, I had the choice of which school I wanted to attend. I ended up staying close to home in Chicago, mainly because we had such a close family. With one dream a reality, it was time to aim for another. When I entered college, I dreamed of starting my own airline. If you are going to dream, you may as well reach for the stars, right? I enrolled in business classes at one of the top schools in the country and signed up for aviation courses. I was in control of my destiny!

Then, at the age of twenty, my self-confidence took a major hit and my life spun into a fast downward spiral. I had a falling out with my college coach, and I didn't know how to put it behind me. This soon led to not having sports in my life, and I lost the structure I was not only used to but also desperately needed. I experienced this desperation with fear because sports and faith in my coaches had been at the center of my life from a young age. My sense of security disappeared, and the foundation I had built my life on crumbled in front of me. To complicate the situation, I made a series of bad choices that eventually landed me in a counselor's office, unable to see which move I should make next.

My life was empty. I tried to fill that void with alcohol and drugs, but that just put me into a deeper depression. I felt unwanted, thinking it might be better if I just disappeared.

Through deep reflection, I decided it was best for me to drop out of school and choose some new scenery. Hopefully the grass on the other side would be greener. However, when I looked out the window of my soul, all I saw was brokenness and shattered glass. The worst part was that I had no idea how to pick up all the pieces. As I drove away from school for the last time, I only saw regret and ill-advised choices in the rearview mirror.

Hitting rock bottom forced me to consider options I said I would never pursue. I was so desperate for a change that I started considering things I had promised myself I would never do. I changed my major to education and transferred to the same small Christian school my parents and grandparents had attended. Talk about a major blow to my ego. I went from having my entire future planned out to sleeping on a dirty couch in my younger brother's dorm room as I waited for classes to begin. Until the semester started, I took the elevated train back and forth to Chicago every day to my part-time accounting job on Michigan Avenue. This daily trek was necessary because paying for college was now my new unfortunate reality. But the only time people were happy in that office was when money came in, and I couldn't imagine one more day staring at a computer screen as I crunched numbers. When I started the semester, I left that position and never looked back.

In April 2002, near the end of my first semester, I had an encounter I would never forget. My brother Joel was dating a girl who I thought was completely wrong for him. I never saw eye to eye with her about anything. As far as I was concerned, she even breathed wrong. His girlfriend repeatedly tried to set me up with her best friend from a middle-of-nowhere farming town in central Illinois. What did people do there besides watch the corn grow?

I had just moved from the fast-paced Lincoln Park neighborhood in Chicago and was not at all interested in meeting anyone from a slow-moving farming community in the boonies. The change of pace from Chicago to the suburbs already felt like I was living in the country. You didn't even have to hurry across the street. After repeated begging from Joel's girlfriend, I finally gave in and agreed to meet her friend from home, mainly because I wanted her to get off my back.

When Joel's girlfriend and her friend Carrie entered the dorm room, I was proven wrong. She was one of the most gorgeous young women I had ever seen! The minute Carrie left the dorm floor, I told all the other college-aged, testosterone-filled guys who were checking her out to keep their distance. I told them to sit back and take notes because Carrie was going to be mine. Obviously I hadn't lost all of my confidence. That day—April 27, 2002—was the last day I wanted to be a free man. In an instant, I immediately changed my opinion about my brother's girlfriend.

Some nights, Carrie and I would meet and stay up playing card games and talking. The dorms had visitation rules—men and women couldn't be on the floor of the opposite sex after the specified times, so we would just hang out in the stairwell between the floors. My unstructured life began to have some structure to it, and I started to respect the values of the Christian school that I now attended. My attitude was changing, whether I wanted to admit it or not.

However, when the new semester started, I resumed my partying lifestyle without her. But at the same time, I couldn't stop thinking about this beautiful girl. Carrie had strong feelings about the type of guy she wanted to date—I might as well have called them "requirements." Let's just say I didn't fit her ideal mold. Having a mouth like a sailor and drinking like a fish didn't impress her, so I started to clean up my act. I cared too much about what she thought not to make adjustments.

Our relationship was growing, and by the next school year, Carrie decided to transfer to my college. We continued to enjoy each other's company and grew closer together as time went on. Then, about a year into our dating life, I started to notice some slow changes in my health that, over time, could no longer be ignored. I was fatigued more often than usual, sometimes even wanting to go to bed at six o'clock in the evening. My normal outgoing personality turned dry and dull, especially evident in my lack of desire to hold a conversation. When I met a childhood friend of Carrie's for the first time, she was so unimpressed that she encouraged Carrie to find someone else to date.

People who knew me well understood that this apathy was a drastic change to my lifestyle. My days of twenty-mile runs and running the midfield during a ninety-minute soccer match were no longer possible. My twenty-one-year-old body was rapidly beginning to break down. Inside I felt like I was dying for an entire year, but no one could figure out what was wrong. Trip after trip to the doctor's office brought me nothing except another misdiagnosis and a growing stack of medical bills. Each trip ended with the same results—more pain medication and more masked symptoms. In times of deep reflection, I thought to myself that I might as well start digging my own grave—my funeral would be coming soon. My fears were growing rapidly into giants I didn't know how to slay.

During this time, I decided to move back home to focus on my health. I continued school and leaned on Carrie for support. The nights were endless. I could really notice my hip bones throbbing when I tried to sleep, pulsating like they had their own heartbeat. I would lie awake in agony for what felt like forever, occasionally arising to pace around my bedroom in an attempt to shake off the pain. If I did fall asleep, the rest was brief, interrupted repeatedly by night sweats. I would wake up, take off my soaking wet clothes, dry off with a towel, and put on something different to wear. I repeated this process four or five times each night for nine months. It grew old very quickly.

Fast forward to January 2004. In a rare burst of energy, I agreed to play in an indoor soccer game where I tripped on the carpet, fell over, and snapped my collarbone in two. It was the first time I had ever broken a bone. The pain meds for the broken collarbone covered up all the other symptoms I was having at the time. Once I was off the pain meds for my collarbone, another diagnosis came for the pain I felt in my hip. My doctor suspected I had a problem with my sciatic nerve, so he prescribed more pain meds as well as muscle relaxers. I was pale, had no appetite, and thought I was going to die before anyone truly figured out what was wrong with me.

I had grown accustomed to incorrect diagnoses, and once again I was discouraged when additional pain medication was prescribed. I was completely out of options, not to mention fatigued, lonely, and fearful for my life. No one understood! I started to think something was wrong with my brain. *Was I imagining all of this?*

Toward the end of January, I student taught in a fourth-grade classroom. This completed one of my last graduation requirements to become a teacher. I remember thinking to myself at the end of my first day, *How in the world can it be this difficult to be a teacher? I know I wasn't attentive in college, but it seems as if there's no way I'll have enough energy for this type of work.*

Twenty-eight nine- and ten-year-olds were now my responsibility.

Somehow I made it through. In April, I was asked to interview for a teaching position for the next school year. As I headed toward the interview, I wondered, *Why on planet Earth would they want me to interview for this position? How in the world could I take care of a classroom of fourth graders when I was struggling to take care of myself?*

In the midst of the ongoing pain from my hips throbbing all day—with no relief gained by sitting, standing, or walking—the principal let me know I was hired as the fourth-grade teacher. I figured I should be excited, but I was too overwhelmed with worry about my health to feel an ounce of satisfaction.

Despite my feelings, I signed the paperwork and accepted the position.

I hit my greatest setback in the middle of April. I was home from school with a fever for an entire week. My already swollen lymph nodes had multiplied and increased in size in my neck, groin, and underarms. I only managed to sleep when I was totally exhausted. I went to a surgeon who specializes in these symptoms, and I sat on the exam table while the doctor felt around my neck. My clammy hands gave away how nervous I was to be in that office.

The doctor turned to me and explained that he needed to do a needle aspiration. *In my neck?! No!* I've had a needle phobia ever since I was a young boy. I can even remember crying when I had to have shots as old as the fifth grade. I don't like to watch horror movies, but I felt like I was in one.

Every muscle in my body went tense as the doctor stuck the long needle into my neck to extract some fluid. I could feel it being sucked from the side of my body into my neck and through the long needle. The doctor drew out so much fluid some of it spilled onto the floor. I was acutely aware that my neck should not have that much fluid! The doctor peered at the nurse with a concerned look on his face. The entire situation played out in slow motion in front of me.

Never in my wildest dreams did I expect to hear what the doctor told me next: "Phil, I've been practicing as a surgeon for over thirty years, and I've seen a few similar situations. There's a fifty percent chance this is cancer." *Cancer?* The c-word threw me into terror. I went into panic mode, and I don't remember anything the surgeon said after that. I imagine they told me they were going to test the sample and call me when the results came in. As I walked out of the surgeon's room that day, my entire existence flashed before me. *If it is cancer, I'm guessing it's advanced—there may not be anything they can do at this point because whatever has been going on has been killing me for a year now.*

The next day I anxiously waited for the phone to ring. *Did I have cancer? Would they figure out what was wrong with me? Could I finally get help? Did I even want to know how bad it was?*

The phone finally rang, and my heart suddenly started to beat faster. It was the doctor. "Phil, we ran the results, and they're negative. It isn't cancer, though at this point I'm not sure what it is." Believe it or not, instead of feeling relief, I felt completely defeated. *Was I going to die before anyone figured out what had gone so terribly wrong?* An entire year of trips to see different doctors, and I still had no answers. The doctor decided it would be best to have a few lymph nodes surgically removed for a biopsy to figure out what was going on.

I had no idea how I was going to get through having surgery. I was deathly afraid of needles and wasn't too crazy about being operated on either, and now I was preparing to go under anesthesia while someone cut into me. My mind went everywhere. Although I knew I should just take things one step at a time and not jump to conclusions or worst-case scenarios, I couldn't stop myself. Having a strong will and great tenacity had worked well for me in the past when I was in control. This was different—now I had to put my fate in someone else's hands. I'm not sure what paralyzed me more—letting someone else operate on me or the idea of facing the unknown.

After my surgery, I went home to rest per doctor's orders. As I waited to find out my fate, I became pensive, reflecting on how unpredictable life could be. Just one year ago, I couldn't have been more optimistic about my future. I was enjoying college life, actively participating in sports, hanging out with friends, and dating the girl of my dreams.

Now, I'd discovered that life could change on a dime and ordinary experiences could become precious rarities. I lay awake in my bed in agonizing pain, looking pale as a ghost, weighing thirty pounds less, with my hips throbbing endlessly. I was completely immobilized by fear—aware that what was coming next could change the course of my life forever.

Reflection Questions

1. Has there ever been a time when you feel like you hit rock bottom? How did you make it out? What questions and decisions in your life did it bring up that you wouldn't have thought about otherwise?

2. Have you ever had to just wait for answers for something that could change your life? What did it feel like to have no control?

CHAPTER 2

PERSEVERANCE

❧

As an athlete, I learned that patience and perseverance can get you through difficult challenges. If you're a runner, you know that the week leading up to any big competition, training tapers down and you focus on eating well, sleeping well, and preparing yourself mentally for the race. When you step out on the track, it's your moment to shine. Your nervous energy is in overdrive and your endorphins kick in.

I found myself in that exact place four years in a row when I competed in the state high school track championships. By the time I stepped on the track for the 800-meter event my senior year, I had run the race a hundred times in my head already. When the gun went off, I took off as fast as possible to get near the front of the pack, paying careful attention not to get boxed in between my competitors and the inside rail. Pushing was normal and necessary as each runner fought to get position.

I knew I had to run a smart race because this was a once-in-a-life-time opportunity. It didn't matter where I was ranked at the start of the race—I could only win with patience and perseverance, running wisely, and performing under pressure. I'll never forget losing that race to a kid in a purple uniform by just a tenth of a second. I learned the hard way that when you lay everything out on the line, sometimes your best just isn't good enough—a timely lesson I was afraid would take hold as I waited anxiously for the most important phone call of my life.

It's amazing the thoughts that ran through my head at that time. It was as if the stock market crashed and all my investments went down with it. My patience was taxed as I waited to see how badly I was hemorrhaging. The ticker-tape inside my head scrolled through an unending narrative that predicted my impending doom. *What if I did have cancer after all? Was it too advanced to treat? What if no one in the medical field could come up with the right diagnosis?*

What if the diagnosis was incorrect again, like numerous times before? Would they only find out what was so severely wrong by doing my autopsy? Today's news would dictate the direction of the rest of my life, and I hated having my life hanging in the balance. I was on edge, waiting to learn if I would have to plan my funeral service or if something could be done to treat whatever was attacking by body. I was drowning in my own worry and anguish.

I stared at the phone next to me, bitter that I had to wait for a call I really didn't want to receive. I didn't know if the news from the doctor would lift me up with joy or crush all my hopes. Fear was suffocating me. I was so filled with terror I wasn't sure if I'd even have the courage to pick up the phone if it did ring. Suddenly, I remembered that my family and I had decided the doctor would call my dad with the results so I could get some rest. Maybe the anesthesia had made me forget, but I took advantage of this realization and fell into a deep sleep.

In the middle of a terrifying dream, I woke up to see my dad sitting at my bedside. Startled, I looked over at the clock—it was only 2:00 p.m. It dawned on me that he must have talked with the doctor. Half-awake, I sat up. *What was he going to tell me? What did he know?* The news could change the course of my life forever. I knew I hadn't done anything wrong to bring on my health issues, and yet I feared that I was about to hear a death sentence. My dad looked me in the eyes as I lay there. He began to speak softly to me.

"Phil, I'm not sure how to tell you this." He let out a long pause. Life seemed to stand still in that moment. The silence was oppressive. He went on gently, "I talked to the doctor, and you have cancer."

"What?"

"You have cancer," he repeated compassionately.

"Dad, are you sure?"

"Yes, Phil. I wouldn't tell you something this serious unless I was sure."

There it was, that dreadful c-word. *Cancer? Me? Now? How could this be? What do I do now?* I knew that a diagnosis was a possibility, but now it was a reality.

We paused for a moment, absorbing the information in silence. Meanwhile, my mind went for a run through all types of terrain. *Am I going to die? I probably need to plan my funeral.* But then I thought, *I have had cancer for a long time with so many symptoms. God has kept me alive so far.* Incredibly, I even felt some relief! We can finally move forward with a course of action. Now at least I knew that the pain I had been experiencing was real—I wasn't just imagining it.

In that moment I went from an undoubtable feeling of desperation to gaining a thimbleful of hope. When you finally know the problem, there must be some solution—theoretically at least, right? There must be something they can do! I tried so hard to be optimistic, though I wasn't fully successful.

Looking back, I imagine my dad never thought he would have to give his twenty-two-year-old son news that would absolutely crush him. Nobody should have to hear those devastating words—words that send you desperately looking for an oxygen tank when it takes your breath away. I wish the three excruciating words "You have cancer" never had to be uttered. I wish no one ever had to hear such news. But the reality was that I had heard those words, and so had millions of others. In order to move forward, I knew the best I could do was to find hope.

Somehow.

I thought about my little cousin Erik. Throughout my life he was the only person close to me who had experienced cancer. He was diagnosed at age four, and unfortunately, cancer took his young life when he was only six years old. Seeing someone so close to me journey through a battle with cancer had made a lasting impression on me. I didn't understand it much, being only two years older than him at the time, but I do recall that the treatment made him really ill.

One of the last memories I had of that experience was when my cousins and I drew pictures for Erik and placed them in his casket at the funeral. Cancer took a terrible toll on that family, and soon thereafter, his parents divorced. Cancer messes with human lives in ways we can never understand or anticipate. *Was I next? Would I die from cancer too? Would those closest to me be torn apart from each other just as it happened in Erik's family?*

As my eyes glazed over in shock, my dad continued to talk. "The doctors say it's Hodgkin's lymphoma." I had never heard of it. He continued to explain that this meant the cancer was in my lymph nodes. As we sat together in quiet desperation, he did the best he could for me in that moment—he prayed. "God, I know that Phil is your child, and whether he lives another month, year, or fifty years, it is my prayer that, through this journey, he can be a witness to you and all that you have done for us."

***

Throughout my life, my determined preparation and self-confidence had come through for me time and time again. Yet, I felt no certainty whatsoever about moving forward in my battle with cancer. I had no experience with this disease to lean on and no idea of how my body would respond to the treatments that were to come my way. I didn't know if I would get through this ordeal or if I would be able to live up to the nightmare I was about to face. In no way was I prepared for what the future held.

How often had I heard the proverbial phrase, "Patience is a virtue" before? With this new diagnosis, I etched out a new meaning for this small, innocuous expression. Knowing myself well, I understood in that moment that my patience would be pushed to its limits during this—the biggest challenge I would ever undertake.

Really, I needed more than patience—I needed perseverance. The simple definition of perseverance is "the ability to not give up." Our ability to persevere is one of the most important tools we can have in our toolbox, and it will, no doubt, directly affect our rate of success in all aspects of life. Navigating a disease like cancer or supporting someone who is fighting this battle really reveals the importance of perseverance.

When I think back to the state track and field championships my senior year, the most important lesson I learned about perseverance came after the 800-meter run. After finishing the race, I fell to my knees out of breath and on the verge of throwing up and passing out. I gave everything in me that I had to give! When I got up to "walk it off," my heart was still running the race. Just two events later was the finals for the 1600-meter run, which I was signed up to participate in as well. I was prepared to scratch the event because I didn't have anything left to give. But my dad encouraged me to go out for it anyway. He saw the persevering qualities in me that I wasn't yet fully aware I possessed. When the gun went off, I dug in as deep as I could. I ran a smart race, and in the final hundred meters, I edged out a few runners and found myself standing on the podium. Once again, I learned that when all odds are stacked against you, the depth of your perseverance can pull you through.

For someone who isn't an athlete, it's easy to think physical shape is the biggest contributor to optimal performance. In reality, it's mental toughness. There's an old adage that says, "Running is ninety percent mental and the rest is physical." I don't know a single runner who would refute this quote. In the same way, when someone journeys through cancer, they immediately think about the importance of their physical health and the toll the cancer will take on their bodies. Physical health can't be discounted in the life of a cancer patient, but one of the biggest tolls cancer can take on a person is on their mental state while fighting this battle. Just like when you're running a race, perseverance is the most important tool in your toolbox when the going gets tough. If you're fighting cancer, you will at times think you can't, but—have no fear—during those times, you may see someone close to you reach out and say with confidence, "Oh, yes, you can!"

Reflection Questions

1. Have you ever given your all for something, but it just wasn't good enough? How did that make you feel? What were the consequences? How did you pick yourself back up?

2. Think of a time when you've needed perseverance to get through something, or something you need perseverance for in your life today. How did you or can you find the strength you need? What form did it or should it take—mental preparation, an encouraging friend, meaningful words, support from a mentor?

PERSEVERANCE

CHAPTER 3

COURAGE IS NOT THE ABSENCE OF FEAR

❧

Just hearing the word "fear" spoken aloud can trigger something from the depths of our soul. We may not even know what we're fearful about when we hear the word, but the very fact it's stirred up something within is a smoke signal sent to us from afar. At times we can write it off as a fleeting thought and nothing significant because, thankfully, that's all it really is.

Unfortunately, we can't always discount fear. When it's real, our senses become intensely heightened and our natural instinct is to scream for it to stop. Fear has tendencies to exaggerate reality and puts an unnecessary emphasis on the unknown, supplying us with a gripping sense of suffocation. Without warning, the internal fire alarm goes off and the panic within is immediately uncontrollable. We could try to ignore it but realize in an instant that never gets rid of it. In our panic, fear is cemented firmly on our face. Our heart quickens and soon the unstable, queasy feeling circulating throughout our body settles deep within every fiber of our being.

Self-awareness can be key to remaining healthy when fear has invaded your spirit. Soon others close to you may become keenly aware of your tormenting fear and detect what's happening even before you notice there's a problem brewing. Still, while enveloped in the fire, your ability to make sound decisions diminishes and in desperation you grab onto anything in your path to alleviate the problem. Eventually, you realize that your attempt to hold on to something is short lived, and you're left with nothing but your feeble attempt at being courageous in the moment.

Nelson Mandela is quoted as saying, "Courage was not the absence of fear, but the triumph over it." I wanted nothing more than to own this sentiment. But after hearing the devastating news, with limited cognitive awareness of what was happening to me, I found it difficult to consider what it would take to move beyond the grips of fear.

In my current state of mind, I continued to try to be hopeful; however, the fear factor was competing for my attention. I learned in that moment that I would be going to battle against a formidable beast on a moment-by-moment basis. I needed time to absorb this information and get some clarity. My dad and I decided to walk a few blocks to a downtown restaurant and grab a bite to eat. On the walk over, random thoughts continued to flood my mind: *How would I break the news of my cancer to Carrie, the woman I envisioned spending the rest of my life with? How would I inform my mom, my brother, and my two younger sisters? What about my principal who was expecting me to teach at the school next year? What about the twenty-eight students I currently taught as a student teacher, all of whom I had grown to love?* I felt heavily burdened by the news of my disease, but almost more burdened with the task of telling the people I loved.

So many individuals had known for such a long time already that I was ill, and everyone in my little world would want to know the latest news. This entire situation had already exhausted me. It's a horrible feeling to be on unfamiliar terrain in the middle of the woods at night, and that's how I felt. It was a struggle to look outside of the circumstances I found myself in. I dreaded the thought of what would happen next and knew in my heart that it would be unpleasant and painful, perhaps even fatal. Deciding who and when and how to tell only added to the difficult challenge. I didn't want to overlook anyone who deserved to hear the news from me personally, but putting together that mental list of people was exhausting and stressful. So many decisions had to be made right away, and I just didn't have the energy or the wisdom to make them. The last thing I wanted to do was field questions. I couldn't imagine getting involved in exhausting conversations about my diagnosis when I hadn't had adequate time to process the news myself yet. I quickly realized there was a short list of people I needed to tell. They needed to hear the news directly from me just as much as I needed to communicate the news personally to them. Anyone else who needed to know would have to find out from others in my family.

After talking through the situation, my dad and I decided on an action plan. I would tell Carrie first. Then that night, when my whole family was home, I would deliver the news to them. Later in the week, I would go to the school and tell my principal and the fourth graders that I had, unfortunately, already taught my last day.

When we arrived back home, I received a phone call from a doctor who was affiliated with a top-ranked cancer hospital. I wondered why he was calling or how he even knew about my situation. It turned out that he had heard from a friend of his that I had received a cancer diagnosis, and he offered to examine my test results. I was aware that a second opinion is usually good, so I accepted his offer and thanked him for calling. I hung up the phone and looked at my dad. I was so caught off guard that it took me a minute to process what had just happened. He was able to connect the dots for me. Earlier that day, he'd reached out to a good friend of his whose daughter had received a similar diagnosis a few years earlier. His friend searched long and hard to find the very best doctor for his daughter. It appeared that this man's hard work could pay big dividends for me. I learned a valuable lesson that day: it's always good to reach out to people you trust when you need help. And it is especially important when you're dealing with life-or-death situations!

It came time for the difficult task of calling Carrie to tell her the awful news. It wasn't ideal to tell her over the phone, but I wasn't going to be able to see her face to face until that evening, and I wanted her to hear the news right away. I couldn't leave anyone in the dark for much longer. I started to shake when I picked up the phone. Telling the woman I wanted to marry that our lifetime together might be cut short, or at the very least would look different than we both had envisioned, was my worst nightmare. I delivered the devastating news and the phone went silent. I'm sure Carrie didn't know how to react to the information, just as I didn't know how to react to her silence. I was so full of emotion that I could hardly think at all. *Was this situation real or was I just imagining all of it? Someone, anyone, come quickly, put your hands on my shoulders and shake me. I need to wake up from this nightmare!* We decided she would come over that evening to be with me after I shared the news with my family.

Then came time to break the news to my family. Again, there was no good way to start this conversation, so I just bit the bullet and went for it. Both of my sisters immediately started crying, and it wasn't long before my mom, dad, and brother had all joined in. My sisters thought their older brother was going to die, and that was more than they could handle. It wasn't like a sports competition, where you know how long the period of play is going to be. In this situation, nobody knew how long the game was going to last or how it would end. None of us knew what the future held. Minutes later, Carrie walked through the back door. There was no doubt what conversation had just taken place.

We all eventually retreated to the family room. I was emotionally exhausted and not up for talking much. My family was in a state of shock and I was too numb to feel anything. To distract us from the emotions that were front and center in our minds, we turned on the TV and attempted to watch a movie. As we were watching, or pretending to, word spread quickly to family and friends about my diagnosis. I told my parents if a call came for me they were to take a message. I didn't want to talk to anyone.

Over the next few hours, the phone rang continuously. Each time it rang, my mom or dad would answer it and go into the other room to take the call. Afterward, they would come back into the room to let me know who had reached out. With a blank stare, I made brief eye contact with my parents but didn't vocalize one response. Instead, I would nod my head to acknowledge what they said and then turn back toward the movie. I looked at the screen, hoping it would provide me with much needed distraction, but it didn't work. I felt as if I was in a dense cloud, and I couldn't see or move or respond to the people around me. I was in a deep, dark cloud of despair. And with my entire family in the same room, I saw on each of their faces this dark cloud as well.

Watching a movie with my family was new to me. It wasn't normal for me to just sit and let the moments tick away—I was always on the go. Some might say I have a short attention span, others that I'm easily bored or just flat-out impatient. I was always on the go because something needed to be done or someone needed to be led. But this pattern of being in complete control was slowly slipping away from me. I didn't like feeling that way and certainly didn't like sitting in this agonizing physical and emotional pain.

Later that night, the phone rang once again. My mom picked it up and began to walk out of the room. Just as I was going to space out of the conversation, she turned around and walked back to hand me the phone. As she did, I thought to myself, *Mom, what are you doing? We had an agreement!* She told me it was the doctor from the University of Chicago.

The uneasy feeling inside me grew ten times worse than I thought possible. Dr. Nachman from the University of Chicago confirmed that I did, indeed, have cancer and asked how long I'd had the symptoms—the night sweats, hip pains, and fevers.

"Nine months," I said.

He informed me that these were signs of stage 4B—the most advanced stage of the disease. I couldn't speak. It was hard to breathe as the devastating news started to take hold and strangle me.

The doctor continued to talk. I caught that he wanted me to come in first thing in the morning to see him. Tears slowly began to stream down my face. I was on the verge of hyperventilating. I did my best to muster the word "goodbye."

One phone call changed my perspective on life as I knew it and I realized that no part of life as I imagined it was promised. After I hung up, I could barely see through the steady stream of tears pouring down my face. I was on the verge of erupting. All this emotion had to go somewhere. I walked into the other room with my head down, unable to hide my anguish. I slowly made my way back to where I was watching the movie on the couch. I turned to look at my family to tell them the devastating news, but the words weren't there. An uncontrollable sobbing took its place. Even though my family tried to console me, I cried and cried and cried. Eventually, I was able to string the words together. "The doctor said I . . . have . . . had . . . symptoms of the . . . most advanced stage of the disease. For probably . . . nine months."

At this point everyone in the room knew and feared the worst. This might be it for me. I sobbed for an hour and only stopped due to sheer exhaustion. The perplexing emotions that had been stuffed down so deep for such a long time had finally come to the surface. My shirt was soaked, my pants were soaked, my eyes were red, and I was too exhausted to feel anything more or even keep my eyes open.

Later that evening, my dad took me aside and handed me a stack of emails he'd printed out over the course of the day. I needed to be alone to read them, so I went down to the quiet basement, sat at a desk and read them one by one. The letters were from people I saw regularly as well as my dad's coworkers, concerned family members, and distant friends. Many wrote words of encouragement, shared a comforting Bible verse, or offered a heartfelt prayer. Others explained how they had followed my health journey and how much my family and I meant to them. They offered their support and commitment to it in the future whenever a need arose.

It was reassuring to know I wasn't going through this awful experience alone, and in that moment I discovered what it truly meant to love one another. I shed a few more tears as I read each email, slowly absorbing the significance of it all. That night, I began to learn how powerful encouragement would be on my cancer journey. In those reflective moments, I realized that these messages of solidarity were sent to show me that I was not going to battle alone. I knew right then and there that those emails needed a place of permanence, so I used them to cover the walls in the corner of the basement where I sat. In times of desperation, I thought, I could go to that little space and be refueled with words of encouragement.

Nature has a way of showing us how important it is that we connect to one another. Take the giant redwoods in California, for example. They are the oldest and largest trees in the world, and one might assume they have root systems that stretch deep into the earth. But their root systems are quite shallow. You might wonder how they can stand firm for such a long period of time. The secret is that the giant redwoods have interconnected roots, so they can help each other remain strong and enduring. Similarly, the support in those email messages that I plastered on my basement walls provided me with the strength and courage I needed to face my fears.

Reaching out to others can help you get through the suffering and anguish brought on by the fear and can turn out to be a tremendous system for coping during those dark moments. For this reason, it is vitally important to seek out others throughout your journey. When you can't see clearly, others can see for you. And their encouragement can bring out the very best in you, pulling you through the ordeal one small step at a time.

Reflection Questions

1. Have you had a time when you needed others' encouragement to get you through a devastating time?

2. How can you be an encouragement to someone you know is suffering? It can be as little as a quick email or phone call, but your encouragement might be just what they need to make it through the next day.

COURAGE IS NOT THE ABSENCE OF FEAR

CHAPTER 4

ENOUGH IS ENOUGH

◈

We live in a digital era. Facts, figures, and opinions are thrown at us in every direction. Opinions are disguised as facts and facts sound like opinions. What if I told you that children in school have longer school days, but less time for physical education and art, and this can have harmful effects? Would you believe me? In your mind, is it an undisputed fact or do you hold the sentiment that it is the opinion of one? Do you need to sift through the research to have an informed point of view?

In our fast-paced world, we get information thrown at us in every direction. As a result, we make quick assumptions and decisions based on what we've heard and don't always discover the truth for ourselves. If we're not cautious, it's possible to trust blindly and, in some cases, find trouble that only compounds later.

We don't have to seek out information—it has a way of finding us: when we get our mail, turn on our TVs, sit at our computers, pick up our handheld devices, get in our cars. Scrolling through social media releases enough dopamine to keep our brains occupied for hours. All this information leads to sensory overload.

I certainly felt as though my brain was on overload—like a transformer that blows up because it receives too much electricity—while I fought the panic that was taking over my body and mind. Now that I knew my diagnosis, I needed to decide how to manage the profusion of detailed information that was going to come my way. I felt like the warning signal in my mind could be heard from a mile away. Overwhelmed? Absolutely! Scared? Definitely! Not knowing what to expect? Undoubtedly! My cancer fight was about to begin, and I had no way of knowing how it would end.

Morning finally came, and my dad took me to the hospital. I was in so much pain, I could barely endure the car ride. Not up for conversation and not knowing what to expect upon arrival, I sat in silence for the entire ride. I knew the hospital was large enough to be considered a small city. My mind started to wander as I thought about what was really inside those four massive walls—the sounds (PA pages, beeping machines, multiple voices talking at the same time), the sights (scurrying nurses, patients hooked up to numerous IVs, bright lights), and the smells (antiseptics, medicines, soiled garments). A sense of foreboding suddenly hit me, and I knew that this crazy environment that was supposed to help me could easily put me over the edge and cause more stress inside my weakened body.

On that first day, like other days that would follow, it was difficult to find a parking spot. We faced the brutal reality that many people face each day—navigating the overwhelming size of the hospital campus to get to the correct destination. When we finally arrived at the right building, it was yet another challenge to find the exact location of my first appointment.

The experience was almost like the first day of high school. It took time to get used to my new surroundings. Figuring out the confusing hallways without seeing familiar faces was intimidating. After repeatedly gazing at my schedule, we anxiously raced around the massive building trying to locate my first appointment. When we finally did arrive and took a seat, my heart was racing. I nervously triple-checked the schedule to confirm I was in the correct location. Like a freshman on his first day of school, I couldn't hide that my confidence was lacking.

A sea of oncology patients of all ages surrounded me in the waiting room. Most of us were there for the very same reason and each of us had to anticipate what was to come next. They call it the "waiting room" for a reason. I tried as hard as I could to not envision a worst-case scenario, but my ever-present fears refused to subside. I already knew I had classic "white coat syndrome," which causes patients to have higher blood pressure than normal when at a doctor's office, even for a routine visit. For me, on that day, the experience was a thousand times worse than usual.

The waiting room was designed with soft colors meant to help patients relax. Fancy tropical fish were swimming in expensive saltwater tanks. The colors and decor offered peace and tranquility, but the anxious faces I saw as I looked around caused the antithesis of what the waiting room environment was to create. I gazed at worn-out faces with large, discolored bags under their eyes, shiny bald heads that showed the side effects of treatments, and bodies that I could tell ached from head to toe. I could literally see the toll this arduous disease had on their body.

When the nurse called my name, I stood up, looked at my dad, and took a deep breath, anticipating what was to come. I locked eyes with the nurse and walked toward her. I could feel the inquisitive eyes of each individual in the room. I was sure they were thinking about how young and healthy I looked—wondering what I was there for. Some probably felt empathy for me, while others were perhaps too tied up in their own anxieties to do so.

After my vital signs were taken, the nurse asked a series of questions

I was unsure how to answer. The questions weren't difficult, but I was in such shock I felt like a preschooler who couldn't understand what was happening. After the initial checkup, I was led to the doctor's office to meet my nurse practitioner and doctor face to face for the first time. More waiting and more anxiety! I was beginning to catch on to the pattern: hurry up and wait.

The experience brought up memories from when I was eight years old and we had some serious renovations going on in our house. It didn't take me long to learn, even at that young age, that construction projects rarely go according to schedule. You have to wait for the foundation to be poured before the framing can begin, electrical work can't start until the framing is complete, etc. Nobody likes undertakings that drag on. Waiting to progress to the next phase felt somewhat like being stuck in a crazy holding pattern until everything was in place where you can finally move on.

After meeting with the doctor and nurse practitioner, the remainder of my day was jam-packed with diagnostic tests. There was more waiting to endure. The test results would be in that night, so, with no time to lose, it was decided that I would check into the hospital early the next morning to start treatment. Over a period of twenty-four hours, I went from not knowing the source of my problems to hearing the gut-wrenching news that I had cancer to moving into the hospital, my new "home."

The only preparation required was for me to pack a bag. In the big scheme of things, that shouldn't have been too difficult. I'd had plenty of occasions when packing a travel bag was necessary. However, the difference was that, for a trip, you normally know how many days and nights you'll be gone. I had no idea how long my stay in the hospital would be. The doctor had just told me to pack a bag; the oncology team would provide me the rest of the details the next day.

The next day, full of the ongoing trepidation and anxiety that had set in upon my diagnosis, I finally sat down in a small room with a team of doctors and nurses. This was my oncology team, and I was meeting most of them for the first time. I tried to digest the large quantity of information that was being shared with me; however, some of the vocabulary seemed like a foreign language. Thankfully, they explained the essentials in a way a fourth-grade student could understand. The upshot was that my organ function was nearly perfect. In light of those results and my young age, they decided to be aggressive and give me as much chemo as I could withstand. The protocol was six cycles of chemotherapy to knock the cancer into remission. Each cycle would consist of three days of inpatient chemotherapy followed by one outpatient treatment.

After going over the logistics of the process, the team informed me of the plethora of potential side effects—including my hair falling out around three weeks after I started my treatment. I was also told to expect the possibility of losing control of anything I considered "normal."

Basically, this included everything I took for granted such as walking, talking, sleeping, keeping food down, keeping normal amounts of energy up—my "new normal" list seemed to go on endlessly. As a human being, and especially an athlete, this information was terrifying. The oncology team was very serious but also extremely positive as they explained the entire process. From my involvement with sports, I knew being on a positive team is a key ingredient to success. Negativity was just as contagious as the cancer and could kill the mood of the team, and in a health crisis, I had a hunch that it could change the overall outlook for me as well.

That day I had a series of other tests, including a CT scan, an MRI, and a PET scan. At the end of the day, as if I hadn't been through enough, they performed a bone marrow biopsy and placed a port in my chest through which chemotherapy treatments could be given and blood samples drawn.

To implant the port, they made an incision in my chest and in my neck and inserted a tube into my jugular vein and fed it down to my heart. The port was surgically implanted in my chest and connected to the tube, allowing the treatment to flow easily to my heart, which would then pump the medication through my body by way of the bloodstream.

All in a day's work. Overwhelming? Yes, to say the very least. I went to sleep that night buried in an avalanche of unwelcome thoughts and information that felt like a premonition of things to come. I knew the next day would be another demanding day, and until that time, I tried with all my might not to give in to the sensation. I was exhausted, but I was ready to declare with defiant determination that dwelling on how grand life was for me in the past would do me no good and could lead me down the path of depression. I also knew that negative thinking about what the future could hold had the potential to bring on unnecessary anxiety. In those intense moments, when I felt defeated and like my life was spiraling out of control, I knew the way to find peace was to conquer each exact moment, one at a time.

Reflection Questions

1. Have you ever had to face something difficult where you didn't know how bad it would be or how long it would last?

2. How do you combat negative thinking and focus on just doing the next thing?

ENOUGH IS ENOUGH

CHAPTER 5

FINDING HOPE IN THE MIDST OF FOG

Standing on the shore looking out over the water and seeing fog in the distance is a strikingly beautiful scene. A luminous, bright glow shining from a towering lighthouse sends messages of hope onto the misty sea. Images like this bring about peace and serenity and are often captured in photographs and paintings. On the other hand, an image of a small fishing boat encapsulated by this fog leaves us wondering what might exist beyond our limited view. In obscurity, colors become dulled, clear images turn bleak and grey, and sensations of hopelessness and confusion set in. At times like these, we desperately long to see through the foreboding gloom.

You know that troublesome feeling when you have too much to do? The opposite is having nothing to do and feeling completely bored out of your mind. Both being overwhelmed and being underwhelmed can make a person feel stuck. You sit motionless with a blank look on your face, not fully functioning or focusing on anything. Imagine being stuck like that for days or even weeks. This was the mental state I found myself in as a cancer patient who confronted drastic treatment plans on a daily basis. I was in a constant fog, strung out on heavy drugs that were intended to help me but, ironically, often left me feeling battered and broken from the inside out. If these drugs hadn't been prescribed,

I'm sure they would have been highly illegal in all fifty states.

One morning while lying in bed, I stared out of my hospital room window into thick fog and heavy rain. As I watched the rain slowly drip down the window, I was awestruck at how this view was symbolic of my life. The window was covered with a blanket of heavy mist that the strongest prescription glasses wouldn't enable me to see through. That morning's wretched view became a metaphor for my future.

I would have selected any other path if given a choice. Often it was so quiet that I could hear every little sound permeating throughout the room. The incessant noises of IV pumps and the faint, whistling sounds of the ever-present oxygen tanks along with a staggering number of other medical contraptions that were connected to me were appalling. The crucial medications messed with my body temperature to an extreme. No matter how much the thermostat was adjusted, I either felt too cold or too warm. At times I was covered with heated blankets and still shivered. Still other moments I was so hot I felt like I was in the middle of a fiery furnace and had to throw off every layer that covered me.

A level of fatigue set in that I had never experienced before. Sometimes I was so tired it became extremely difficult to fall asleep. I quickly realized that the rules in the hospital weren't the same as staying overnight at a serene campground. In the hospital, there are no quiet hours. Nurses and doctors would pop in to monitor my vitals, oxygen levels, and medications and run tests on me throughout the night. As if this wasn't frustrating enough, I could hear the constant high-pitched noises of monitors going off in other patients' rooms along with an occasional yell. Throw in a few code blues over the speaker system, and I wondered what on Earth was happening next door. The uncertainty of my neighbor's condition made the uncertainty of my own situation even more frightening. Every time the nurse walked into the room to hang another bag of chemo, the ritual was the same, "What is your name and birth date?" I would give her the response I've given at least one hundred times already, "Phil Zielke, June 26, 1981." The nurse would look at the ID band to confirm this information. She would then proceed to scan the barcode on my wristband and the barcode on each medication to add to my permanent medical file. Finally, it would be time for the last follow-up question, which I knew by memory as well: "Do you have any allergies?" I would always respond the same way, "No, not that I know of." As usual, the questioning portion would end successfully and my chemo treatment would finally be allowed to start. This stringent routine was beyond monotonous.

When my treatment was finished and I received a few blood transfusions, I knew my hopeful discharge date would ultimately be impeded. The round of treatments left my insides unsettled like water boiling on a hot stove. I tried to reposition myself in bed to feel better, but every move left me feeling worse. Again and again, I threw up bile because there was nothing left in my stomach to offer in its place. Each time I rotated an inch in bed or moved my head to the left or to the right, I would vomit once again.

The treatment became so severe it caused nausea to sweep over me like a crashing wave. The normal anti-nausea medication I'd become accustomed to just wasn't doing its job.

Therefore, the medical team attempted to rescue me the only way they knew how. They threw me into a life preserver in the form of a new anti-nausea drug that provided some relief, but had its own array of side effects and challenges that came along with it. As I flitted in and out of consciousness, I remember the nurse vaguely saying to me, "99.9 percent of people do not have an allergy to this anti-nausea drug, so you should have nothing to worry about." I didn't think much of her statement at the time. It was a miracle I even remembered what she said because my short-term memory was functioning at the level of an Alzheimer's patient—another side effect of chemo.

When I finally felt a little better, I was discharged. From experience, I knew that three days of chemotherapy could land me in the hospital for another three-week stay as my body fought its hardest to recover. I was glad to go home, but I knew a simple fever or slight change in my situation would make my discharge short-lived.

When I arrived at home, I started to feel a little better and decided it would be a nice idea to walk around the block with my mom and sisters. I hadn't felt well enough to attempt a walk in weeks, so I knew to capitalize on the moment. As we made it to the cul-de-sac at the end of our street and prepared to make a left turn, I felt some tightness in my chest. *Probably just heartburn,* I thought to myself. However, a short while later my left arm started to tighten. My sisters thought I was joking around, knowing my tendency to prank them.

When we were halfway around the block, my jaw began to lock up and my windpipe started to close as well. I knew something was seriously wrong. As we made the last turn back onto our street, the entire left side of my body went stiff and breathing became an arduous task. Even taking a few steps forward was difficult. In that instant, I doubted I'd be able to make it home without assistance. By the time we returned to our house, my face had turned ashen. By this time, my sisters knew this was no joking matter, and they ran with lightning speed into the house to ask my dad for help.

My dad drove me to the local hospital as fast as he could while I gasped for air. Upon arrival, I staggered like a wounded warrior into the crowded emergency room. If I didn't get help soon, I knew this very well could be the end of my life. My panic-stricken dad explained to the woman behind the desk that I couldn't breathe. She responded that many people were waiting ahead of me, and I needed to wait my turn.

I'm sure that was standard protocol to follow in her position—first come, first served. Had she known the severity of my dilemma I believe she would have assessed the situation differently. My dad pleaded my case to the emergency room clerk begging for any kind of help. But it became clear that I needed to "wait my turn."

During this time, I decided to stagger outside with the remaining strength I had, thinking I might have a better fighting chance if I could breathe in some fresh air. I didn't know what else to do. In the process, I collapsed on the hot blacktop, no longer able to move to the left side of my body. I remember looking up into the blue sky and crying out to God as I lay on the heated asphalt. Angry and disappointed, I prepared to take my final few breaths. I thought to myself, *I made it this far through all those painful treatments. Is it possible I would simply die from an avoidable complication due to anti-nausea medication?* The second that thought crossed my mind, I was rushed into the ER. I was finally admitted thanks to people waiting in the emergency room. They complained to the hospital staff that the kid outside needed help now or he was going to die.

The attending doctor asked me a series of questions, but I lay motionless as I struggled to get any words out. He leaned a little closer to see if that would provoke a response. With the doctor's face now a foot away from mine and a nurse keeping me awake by rubbing her hand through my hair, I somehow managed to miraculously squeeze out a few words: "I had Compazine." Within twenty seconds, I was given an IV shot of Benadryl to reverse the dystonic reaction I was having to the drug, and I could instantly breathe again.

My life flashed in front of me. Finally, I began to cry. As I lay there taking deep breaths, I looked toward my dad and at the hospital staff with tremendous appreciation and thanked the doctors and nurses for saving my life. This experience reminded me that while dealing with this dreadful disease, the quality of my life could change in an instant.

At times, I had the feeling of being stuck and all alone with nobody to turn to. Isolation was very common for cancer patients, but that didn't make it any less difficult. For various reasons, on any given day, I chose not to have visitors. At times I didn't feel comfortable with anyone seeing the hideous shape my body and mind were in. I discovered that some people who cared deeply about me didn't know what to say, so they kept their distance.

People I thought would visit me never did.

When people disappeared and didn't show up during the tough times, it made me wonder if they just didn't care. But over time I came to learn that wasn't it. I believe that, sometimes, the people closest to me kept their distance during my cancer battle because they were nervous and unsure of what to say. But the presence of friends and family members had never mattered to me more. I desperately needed support on this journey. I learned that it was never too late for someone to show up, and it was a great reminder to me that I wasn't forgotten when they did.

Their presence was one of the best gifts they could have ever given me at that time. Sometimes people would travel to see me, but I didn't let them in because I was too ill (even a common cold could put me at risk of death). Even being told after the fact that a visitor had come encouraged me. When friends and family would press their hands on the glass and peek in through the window of my isolation room, I would turn my head to make brief eye contact with them. Although I had no energy to smile or change my facial expression, their presence reassured me that they cared.

All too often spouses leave, families shy away, and friends disappear when the difficult news of cancer comes into the picture. Losing your health is devastating and often sends your life into a downward, out-of-control spiral into financial difficulty and a period of utter ruin. When I was diagnosed with cancer, a number of people close to the situation told my girlfriend, Carrie, to break up with me. They reasoned that she would have to deal with my disease for some time to come. She had her entire life in front of her—why should she let me get in the way of that?

These so-called friends were confident she could find another guy to make her much happier.

Carrie didn't take their recommendations. Instead, she dedicated her life to me. Even while taking twenty credit hours and working at a restaurant on evenings and weekends, she took trips back and forth to the hospital to care for me. On her dinner breaks, we would meet halfway and sit on a park bench overlooking a pond. These consistent visits provided the much-needed pick-me-up I desperately longed for. Thankfully she didn't exit my life and understood the true, persevering nature of love.

***

Even with Carrie and other loved ones by my side, I felt trapped in a dangerous, hopeless place. At times, I felt like I was being buried alive. But during this long journey I discovered that, with the help of others, there was truly reason for hope.

It's easy to feel hopeful and peaceful when looking out from the safety of the shore and only seeing fog in the distance. However, it's a much different story when our position changes and we find ourselves staring directly into the uncertain perils that lie ahead. Facing a life-threatening disease leads to a lot of uncertainty, where feelings of hopelessness can overtake us.

Still, inside this space, it is possible to find hope if we are intentional to look for it. When we discover ourselves in the midst of fog, the colors are grey—but searching for hope can gradually stain our world a brighter color.

Power and clarity of purpose unleash in our mind when we're able to see through the fog, and this is where we find hope that is more beautiful to us than if we had never entered the fog in the first place.

Reflection Questions

1. In your suffering, have you had people show up for you that you didn't expect? Did others not show up who you expected to show up?

2. How can you be there for someone else who is suffering, even if you are nervous or unsure or what to say?

CHAPTER 6

WORDS HAVE POWER

We are designed internally and externally with connecting features that we've come to rely on without even knowing it. Our body organs and tissues work together to carry out important jobs. Trillions of cells with their own specialized functions group together to form organs and blood vessels that are connected to create each body system. A pregnant woman establishes an intimate connection with the life growing inside of her. Teachers connect with students so they can grow into law-abiding citizens, and doctors and nurses connect with patients to show they care about their well-being.

When our bodies are broken and we find ourselves weakened, not only by our physical pain but also by our emotional anguish, we soon discover the situation could be made worse if nobody were available to comfort us during this time of suffering. Many of us take pity on a person when they are down and nobody is there to lift them up. Nothing can replace the power of physical touch along with positive interactions because, as humans, we are designed to connect with one another. When we're sick, strong and healthy connections are necessary and can be life-giving.

My dad often visited me and modeled the type of connection I craved. His typical routine was the same each time he came to see me.

Before entering my room, he would knock, tell me who he was, and slowly open the heavy wooden door. If I felt up to it, I would give him a head nod signaling it was okay to come in, or I would answer aloud to give him permission to enter. He would pay careful attention to the precautions on the door such as washing his hands and putting on the required gown, gloves, and mask. He was also intentional about keeping the stress of his day outside of my room. My dad was so "zoned in" on meeting me where I was that his mere presence ushered peace into my life that I didn't have before he entered my room. It was such a gift!

Some days he didn't have to speak a word because his presence said, "I love you, son. I'm here for you. Whatever I can do, just ask." In my presence, his only agenda was me and this connection was like a much-needed breath of fresh air.

Occasionally, when I had a visitor or was talking with someone over the phone, I wasn't able to communicate effectively. I maintained a slower pace in the conversation because of the overwhelming stress I was facing, and because of that, it frequently took me longer than usual to gather my thoughts and turn them into words. As a result, I discovered that, when a friend or family member visited or called, the single most valuable part of our time together was when they showed active, empathetic listening, no matter how slow and laborious my words were. I wanted the gift of their full presence.

Life in the hospital is a different world, so I appreciated when visitors were thoughtful about slowing down their pace when visiting me. These small adjustments showed me that they cared for me in a big way. On occasion, when a visitor would ask me open-ended questions, it helped me process the myriad of emotions I was dealing with at that moment. Other times, I would start to cry and not even know why.

During my long-term stays in the hospital, I also made connections with healthcare professionals. The first time I interacted with my nurse practitioner it was clear she understood my needs. Kelly would sit next to me, listen closely, and hold my hand. Her presence alone provided me with peace. Each time I spoke with her, it was like talking to an older sister who was looking out for me. To this day, I can recall the deep bond that formed between us and how safe she made me feel while I was going through the greatest hardship of my life.

When I was feeling miserable, I discovered that it was perfectly acceptable to set up boundaries with people who would leave me exhausted. Stress was an impediment to my healing process, and it wasn't unusual for my stress levels to elevate when people didn't take into account what was best for me. I remember a few visitors who entered my room and were as enthusiastic as high school cheerleaders. They meant well, but I didn't have the energy to take part in their cheeriness. I wanted them to tone it down so I could appreciate their visit and get the most out of our time together. We weren't in a high school gymnasium watching a basketball game; we were in my hospital room where I was fighting for my life.

***

While on this journey, time and time again, I experienced firsthand what could happen if someone didn't fully understand the consequences of an unfiltered comment. Words can either breathe life or deflate hope as quickly as a needle popping a balloon. Hurtful comments, even well-intended, were more noticeable to me while I was in this compromised state.

Before getting sick, it was not uncommon for me to be a little unfiltered and flippant when speaking to others. I just said what was on my mind, no matter who I was speaking to or what the situation may have been. But I soon came to realize the importance of speaking the way you want to be spoken to, especially when speaking to someone who is desperately trying to hold onto hope. I quickly learned that these negative and insensitive comments were like smoke coming through an air vent. Early detection was key to ensuring they didn't cloud the view or dishearten the spirit.

Overall, my journey taught me that most people are well-intentioned, but not always cognizant of the effect their words may have. One individual who was very close to me was having a particularly rough day emotionally, but decided to visit me anyway. She said, "Phil, you need to get out of the hospital. Don't you understand this is hard on all of us?" I know she didn't mean to be that aggressive with her comment, but by the time she realized how it sounded it was too late to take it back.

Others would come to visit and tried to fill the void with a common conversation-starter such as, "So, Phil, how are you feeling?" In most situations, this innocuous question could typically be used to get a discussion going. However, it felt unintentional and insensitive when I was hooked up to IVs, getting chemotherapy, attacked by side effects, and feeling like crap all over.

Flippant comments that are typically used in everyday conversations can be extremely hurtful to a sick person. Once I was at home in between treatments, and a few people came over to the house. They were talking about the busyness of life and one man used a phrase I used often before I was sick: "Man, I feel like I'm dying." The words cut into my heart like a knife. I immediately got up from my chair and exited the room. "I feel like I'm dying" is not what you want to hear in casual conversation when you're facing your own mortality.

Don't beat yourself up if you haven't used your words well in the past. You're not alone—it's as common as breathing. A good reminder moving forward is to be sure to check the condition of your heart before you speak. What wells up underneath the surface can pack a lot of heat and, just like a geyser, it will eventually blow. Also, evaluate the situation you're in, especially if you're communicating with someone who is sick. Consider that they may have no more tolerance for toxic interactions.

When we choose to speak with intentionality to make a positive impact, we can unleash enough power to rescue a friend from a pit of despair. However, if we are careless with our words, they can devastate others like a sting of a thousand bees. Give thought to what you're going to say before you speak, and above all, be kind. Remember one comment can have the impact of a thousand words and a thousand words can have the impact of one. Cling to the idea that you have the ability to make a difference for good through the power of your words.

When we visit someone who is sick, it's important to get "zoned in." Friends or family members living with cancer don't need any more stress. So we must do our best to observe the situation, deliberately listen, match their energy levels, and ask open-ended questions that are meant to stimulate conversation and can easily be viewed as an invitation to join in. The time spent together will either help the wounded gain more peace from the visit or remove any semblance of comfort that was there. When living with cancer, a person can't afford to take steps backward when they are in the fight for life, so it becomes vitally important to always consider meeting them exactly where they are.

Reflection Questions

1. When have words breathed life into your situation? When have words caused harm?

2. Have you ever said something with good intentions but it ended up being hurtful? What did you learn from the situation?

CHAPTER 7

STAYING POSITIVE AND EXPERIENCING JOY

⁊

Adiagnosis or loss is a lot to carry and fear can most definitely add to the weight. Now mix fear with a flood of emotions and we're bound to experience a deficit in our decision-making process. As if the intense weight of the situation isn't enough, we are now expected to think clearly and make informed decisions today that may greatly affect our tomorrow while being bombarded with a massive amount of information from all directions.

Our greatest chance of success occurs when we move one step at a time, focusing on slowing down and living in the present. When we practice this on a daily basis, a pathway opens up to improve our ability to make clear decisions. In the process, peace will replace the feeling of being inundated with all the decisions that need to be made.

Slowing down can be challenging at first, but it can also bring big returns in the end. To streamline the process, we first need to protect ourselves from the deluge of information that can become available to us by searching for the truth. Sifting through the abundance of information can be exhausting, but brings confidence as you take your next step.

Choosing to remain positive in my attitude and thoughts was one of the most crucial decisions I made while battling cancer. Staying positive is a daily choice and takes major mental and physical energy to maintain. When I continued to look at the overwhelming picture of my cancer journey, I realized I was setting myself up for failure. So, early on, one strategy I implemented to make my life more manageable was to look at each day as a twenty-four-hour chunk of time.

Even then, sometimes just taking it one day at a time was too much to handle. I sometimes focused on living an hour at a time; other times, I was forced to look at my life in one-minute increments. During my most intense treatments, some of these minutes felt like never-ending hours to me. But being optimistic during these dark moments was a lifeline for me.

It helped to have a support system, not just from friends and family but also from those who really understood what I was going through. Once I attended a party at a friend's house. At one point, the women were hanging out in the living room, and the men were hanging out in the kitchen. It just so happened that all those guys played in the National Football League—that is, everyone except me. Some were longtime NFL veterans who had played in Super Bowls; others had won the NFL's most prestigious awards. To say I felt out of place would be an understatement.

Those guys had a great bond with each other because they had a similar background playing in the NFL. With my limited playing experience—okay, zero playing experience—there was no way I could have had the same camaraderie they shared, especially regarding football. It made sense to me that the deepest bonds were formed with others who shared similar experiences.

In the same way, a group of cancer patients can form strong bonds and deep relationships quickly because of our shared experiences. They have a mutual understanding of what each other is going through. They bond over their journeys as they share stories filled with victory and pain. Cancer patients can quickly form a bond that has the potential to last a lifetime. A person who has not experienced cancer cannot share the same depth of understanding.

Some of the many people I've met on my cancer journey have had a profound effect on my life. I could make a long list of cancer patients I've formed deep bonds with. One such person who would be on that list is a young girl named Jenna. We first met when I was twenty-two years old and she was four. Jenna had her childhood ripped away from her at an early age when she found out she had cancer. Meeting a young child who no longer had free time to play and who felt subpar because of her intense treatments made me think that I was talking to a miniature adult. When Jenna and I were receiving outpatient treatments, we often sat next to each other. One day the nurse came in to get our IVs started and to hang our next bag of chemo. Most adults are not fond of needles, so you can imagine how painful this was for a four-year-old. The nurse gave me my needle first and then turned to Jenna and said, "Look, Phil can do it." Then Mandy, Jenna's life-size doll and her constant companion, received her needle. The nurse again turned to Jenna and said, "Look, Mandy can do it too." It encouraged Jenna to receive her needle as well.

Jenna is now a two-time brain cancer survivor. After Jenna's bout with cancer, her parents decided to forgo having more children of their own and decided to adopt a little girl from China. The family was thrilled about the new addition to their family, especially after all the pain they had been through. Shortly after adopting Abby, they found out she was having pain in her eye. After running tests, the doctors gave the family another devastating blow: Abby had cancer. Fast forward a few years later and now Abby is a two-time cancer survivor just like Jenna. You might think to yourself, *What horrible luck this family has had.* But if you talk with Jenna and Abby's parents, you won't hear them feeling sorry for themselves. One benefit of having cancer is that it gives you a wider perspective on life. If Jenna had never had cancer, they would never have adopted Abby. If Abby was never adopted, the cancer would have never been detected, and Abby wouldn't be alive today. I have a deep bond with this family that has stood the test of time.

Cancer was the bond that brought us together.

Hearing stories of survival never gets old, and thankfully there are many. Unfortunately, over the years, I've also heard many stories that ended in heartbreak. One such story happened years ago when Carrie met Krista. Carrie was sitting in a college class and noticed that Krista had a scar on her chest that resembled the aftermath of a chemotherapy port. Carrie struck up a conversation with Krista and asked her if she'd had cancer. When Krista told Carrie that she did, she wondered how Carrie knew. Carrie responded, "I saw the scar on your chest from your port." She then told Krista that her boyfriend was also a cancer survivor. It turned out that Krista, too, was a Hodgkin's lymphoma survivor, and our birthdays were only a few weeks apart. Krista and Carrie didn't talk much to each other in class that day, but those few words built a bond between them.

Krista's story gets more interesting. Krista ended up student teaching at my school in the classroom next to mine. We formed an instant bond because of what we had both been through. A few years later, Krista was diagnosed a second time with Hodgkin's lymphoma. In her first cancer battle, she'd had a stem-cell transplant using her own stem cells. The second time she was diagnosed she needed a stem-cell donor. Her brother was a perfect match. During the transplant, Krista contracted graft-versus-host disease (GvHD) and, devastatingly, died a short time later.

Krista and I had formed a close bond that helped us both stay positive during our journeys, but cancer brought it to an end. How can

Krista and I have such similar stories and yet such different outcomes? I can't answer that, but I do believe that we don't choose our paths, and somehow we have to trust that all of this is for a higher purpose. What makes this statement difficult to swallow is that we don't always see how all the pieces fit together on this side of heaven. Another friend of mine named Carolyn was looking forward to a much-needed vacation with her husband and two sons, part of her plan to stay positive before a necessary stem-cell transplant. The upcoming transplant, without complications, would keep her in the hospital for a minimum of three weeks. Thankfully all of her counts were good enough for her to go on vacation before the procedure would take place.

The doctor administering her chemotherapy and giving her the green light to travel was filling in for her primary doctor who was on vacation. Through her past experiences with cancer treatments, she knew that her blood counts would take a major dip in the next few days and that would lead to needing a blood transfusion. Leaving the hospital without the transfusion would be like getting in the car without enough gas to make the trip. She would never make her intended destination.

The doctor on call did not understand how her body would respond to the chemotherapy because he hadn't been walking the journey with her over the past year. As a result, he denied her request for the transfusion. However, Carolyn drew a line in the sand and vowed to herself and her family that she would not take no for an answer. She raised a mega-sized stink. Her determination and fight resulted in the doctor changing his decision, Carolyn was able to enjoy her vacation. As the saying goes, "When the going gets tough, the tough get going." To stay positive, sometimes a cancer patient has to fight for their rights and this may mean getting tough and standing strong for their medical and emotional well-being.

We do what we have to do to survive and not give up hope. While others close to me continued to make memories together in the outside world, I stared at hospital walls. I learned an important routine from someone close to me that I followed regularly. It all started on a trip that I took after I finished my cancer treatments. I was waiting for a cab to take me back to the airport after an amazing week spent in Cancun, Mexico. I dreaded returning home to zero-degree temperatures in the middle of a Chicago winter. Reality was about to hit me like a brick, and I was bummed that the vacation I had been looking forward to for so long was about to end.

The person who was on the trip with me suggested I take one last walk out on the beach and capture a mental picture and to remember the image. On that bright and sunny day, I walked out to the beach and stood with the soft sand sinking beneath my feet. I paused for thirty seconds and snapped several pictures in my mind. To this day, I still carry vivid mental images with me, and I take them out when times are rocky and I need to feel peace. Those views took me to a spectacular place, and it cost me nothing.

Some of the most peaceful stored images for me are those where I see myself sitting near my backyard pond listening to the tranquility of the waterfall. When I was well enough to be home, I would take my lawn chair and sit alone by the water enjoying the moment. When it wasn't physically possible to be outside, I would close my eyes to mentally escape to peaceful places. I learned that I needed to do what I could to stay positive by taking myself to pleasant places in my mind's eye. Even today, to stay optimistic during dark moments, I take a picture on my cell phone to view at a later time, but mostly I just enjoy the mental images that I have in my head.

Amazingly, losing my health gave me a great opportunity to find joy, and during my battle with cancer I began to appreciate everything else I'd been given. I would remind myself on a regular basis that I needed to decide to stay positive and choose joy each day. No matter what I was facing, I knew that I could find inexpressible joy and rediscover hope if I made the right choices. I could choose to take a nap, pick up a book, talk with a friend, watch a movie, or go for a peaceful walk. It took me a while, but I soon realized that the more I found reasons for joy in my life, the better I became at finding it.

When an intense situation or trauma—such as cancer—enters our lives unexpectedly, it appears to be only a curse. However, if we dig underneath the surface and through the rubble, we can find blessings that begin to shine like diamonds. By slowing down, even when we're reluctant to do so, we can discover such buried treasure. The slower pace we're forced to move at can heighten our awareness of unhealthy patterns in our lives that may have otherwise gone unnoticed. As adults, we make 35,000 barely conscious decisions each day. As our level of responsibility increases, so does the smorgasbord of choices we face. To exacerbate matters, our fast-paced world doesn't always leave us much spare time to self-reflect and search for the beauty within ourselves and in the people around us. When we are persistent and intentional about slowing down, it's more likely that we will become aware of the value and uniqueness of others. Cancer is a circumstance no one chooses, but a silver lining is that it gives us unavoidable moments to slow down, evaluate various patterns in our lives, and make changes for the better. In the end, each intentional decision we make throughout our day can give us unique opportunities to stay positive while searching for the sweet serenity of joy.

Reflection Questions

1. Is there anyone in your life who "gets" you in a way no one else does because of what you both have been through?

2. What small joys in your life can you choose when you're going through a rough season?

CHAPTER 8

TAKING ADVANTAGE OF AN UNEXPECTED REPRIEVE

Have you ever been on the receiving end of good news? Was it the time when you learned that you and your spouse were expecting a child? Or was it when you heard that you finally got the news that you've been promoted (with a substantial salary increase, of course)? Maybe it was the time you were waiting anxiously until you finally received word that the offer on your dream house was accepted. Good news can come in all shapes and sizes, and when it's delivered, it's as if a dark cloud has been lifted and the beaming sun breaks through.

But none of these joys compare with the words that cancer patients hope to hear: "You are cancer free." Fortunately, due to early detection and advancements in cancer treatment, patients today have a much greater probability of hearing those precious words, which instantly send a flood of emotions from head to toe. The doctor's news should be shouted from the mountaintops. Bring out the champagne and jump for joy! It's time to party! These incredible words make grown men and women cry. Within hours, great joy spreads from caregivers to family to friends. The jubilation is nearly unequaled.

In early September 2004, a PET scan revealed what I had been praying it would show. I heard those wonderful words that caused a flurry of emotion to sweep over my family and me: "Phil, you are cancer free." This was cause for celebration! Carrie, my parents, my siblings, extended family, and friends all celebrated with me.

As I left the hospital upon receiving the incredible news, unbelievable happiness swept over me, especially when I saw the hospital building in my rearview mirror. Unfortunately, I knew that this didn't mean the grim reaper wouldn't continue to pursue me. I also knew what was ahead: a series of scheduled tests that were common next steps for survivors as doctors and technicians monitored me for months and years to come. Each time I experienced an ache or pain that even resembled a hint of how I used to feel, I couldn't help but wonder if I was still in the clear. Fear would creep in like a termite, doing damage before I even realized it was there. But the optimistic side of me believed the nightmare was finally over. I could breathe easy again. I was able to turn the page on this unwelcome chapter in my life.

As I started over with my new identity—a cancer-free man—I took new insights with me along the way. It seemed as if, in a short amount of time, I had experienced a lifetime of knowledge that caused me to establish a new set of priorities. I developed a heightened awareness for my health, my family, and my purpose. After what I had been through, I knew firsthand that tomorrow was not promised so I decided to live each day that did remain with purpose. In my relationships and daily activities I focused on how everything fit into the bigger picture as opposed to letting little things become distractions. I listened to my body and now better understood how my decisions and what was going on in my body affected the way I felt. I let go of negative influences and toxic relationships in my life and replaced those relationships with people who have similar values and a zest for life. I learned to forgive myself more easily, laugh more, and enjoy each moment. It was clear to me that God was in control of my present and my future, so I relinquished control to him and focused on what I was responsible for. I let go of my worries and fears and focused on my purpose and the one who gave me purpose. I desired to share my faith with others and dedicated my time to being a leader and a servant as opposed to following selfish desires. I was present with myself and with my family and whenever I thought to myself how much I loved them, I voiced it. Cancer wasn't an experience I would have chosen to go through, but it produced perseverance, focus, and a healthier, more balanced life overall.

My strength increased each day, but I still wondered if my body would ever physically return to its pre-cancer form. It was difficult to tell in real time, but as the days and weeks went by, positive changes became obvious to me and others around me. Eventually I was able to make it through the day without napping. Soon my motor skills returned to where they'd been before cancer came along, and my quivering hands settled. Once again, I had no trouble using a zipper. My complexion changed back to normal, and my persistent heartburn subsided. My hair came back with a vengeance and was as soft as a newborn baby's. Thankfully, hair showed up on my legs again too, so I no longer looked like I belonged in a skirt. I had to get used to shaving my face again. Plus, my blood count rose to healthy levels, and I was no longer at risk for internal bleeding.

Many of the bodily functions I'd taken for granted prior to cancer also returned. However, my body was scarred from multiple surgeries and I felt geriatric going through the motions of life. The biggest side effect of chemotherapy that still plagues me to this day is malfunctioning salivary glands. Dry mouth is now a regular occurrence. Only those who have gone through this experience can understand what a nuisance this is on a daily basis.

My cancer also adversely affected my dental health, which I had enjoyed and valued ever since second grade when a beloved teacher had emphasized the importance of brushing our teeth. Mrs. Loek greatly influenced my life. I distinctly remember a few things about her that left an indelible impression on my life. She was about four feet tall (I don't think they make teachers that short anymore). And she was about ninety years old (I don't think they let teachers teach that long nowadays). Lastly, she offered frequent advice and provided me with life lessons. It wasn't unusual for this experienced teacher to become frustrated with me for my lack of diligence with my memory work. As if she had a premonition, one day she reasoned with me, "Phil, this memory work you keep fighting me on and don't want to learn will be important to you someday, and it may be a time when you're on your hospital bed and too sick to open your eyes."

Mrs. Loek also preached the importance of brushing our teeth. She was living proof of the value of this type of daily hygiene: even at her age, she'd never had a cavity. I was doing well for years following Mrs. Loek's advice until cancer hit. Chemotherapy ruined my teeth. I visited the dentist after completing treatment only to find one of my teeth had halfway rotted out. The rest of the tooth was drilled out without the help of novocaine (cancer raises your pain threshold!). My pearly whites also faded to a stained yellow. Now, as a cancer survivor, I'm used to brushing my teeth more often and chewing gum. Most importantly, I'm constantly drinking water to help with my perpetually dry mouth.

The chemotherapy wreaked havoc on my prostate and digestive tract as well, and although I didn't look like a cancer patient on the outside, my insides were still scarred in many ways. Have you ever seen those commercials that ask, "Do you have a going problem?" Unfortunately, I did. I had to use the bathroom frequently for months after finishing treatment, to the tune of six or seven times a night.

With the treatments cancer patients endure, it's no wonder they have ongoing health issues afterward. In the war against cancer, my body took a beating. But receiving the treatments and their aftermath was the price I paid for the opportunity to celebrate another birthday. The traumatic long winter of cancer was finally over, and my body was now ushering in the newfound life of spring. I had often wondered if this day would ever come, but now it was here, and I welcomed it joyfully.

Soon I was healthy enough to return to work and start my first year as an educator. The fourth graders were excited about their new teacher. These young students were at an impressionable age, and, for most of them, I was their first male teacher. I started a month late due to my treatment. In addition, my immune system needed to rebound before I entered a classroom full of germs.

Teaching was a difficult transition. I started with a few hours each day, moved to half a day, and eventually transitioned to full-time work. Limited physical stamina slowed me down. Every time my students left for another class, I posted a Do Not Disturb sign on the door, turned off the lights, and passed out on the beanbags inside the reading center. When I forgot to set my alarm or didn't hear it because I was in a deep sleep, I awoke to the clatter of rambunctious nine- and ten-year-olds returning to the classroom. These little bite-sized jolts of energy were sometimes too much for me to handle, but, in the long run, I began to see how they were also crucial for me during the transition process. Their excitement was contagious and helped me enjoy my work even when I was running on empty.

Looking back at that time my life, I see that many of the typical stress points of the cancer journey were taken care of for me beyond my wildest dreams. A variety of people helped me return to work. Kelley, a coworker of mine, drove me to school and Sharolyn, my partner teacher across the hall, took care of lesson planning as well as assisting me in countless ways behind the scenes. I had a long-term substitute teacher,

Diane, who provided stability for my students and always stepped up to fill in when my body hit the wall. It took an army of caring individuals to get me back on my feet again.

During this time I had much to be thankful for. I also had much to celebrate. In February, I made plans to propose to Carrie. Although I was in no way a stellar boyfriend, she had been an unshakable refuge throughout the difficult storm of cancer.

Carrie overwhelmed me in many ways with her numerous examples of unconditional love and devotion. Without her unwavering encouragement and steadfast dedication to seeing me on the road to recovery, I most likely wouldn't be alive today. She missed out on her last summer at home before graduating college and moved into her great-aunt's house in a southern suburb of Chicago to be closer to me. She took on that restaurant job in the western suburbs in order to visit me daily. She practically lived out of her car the entire summer as she went back and forth to the hospital.

When it was time to pop the big question, trepidation set in, but there was no doubt in my mind that I wanted to spend the rest of my life with this woman. I decided to propose in an unexpected way because she always enjoyed a good surprise. For this once-in-a-lifetime experience, I planned to have as many people in attendance as possible, partly because I figured there was a greater chance she would say yes if I asked her in front of others.

I decided the fourth/fifth grade Valentine's Day dance at school would be the perfect opportunity. The dance was a big deal for the kids. In many cases, they brought their moms or dads as dates. The school catered food, brought in a DJ, and sent the kids home with a keepsake photo. I prepared to propose toward the end of the evening. I was sweating bullets even though I tried to think of everything beforehand. My brother, Joel, was there to provide emotional support and to ensure

I didn't misplace the ring. Plus, to savor the moment, Tom, one of my roommates from college, was there to videotape the occasion. With every box checked, I had the DJ publicly ask Carrie to make her way to the center of the dance floor so the fourth graders could honor her in a unique way. A singular chair awaited her as she crossed the threshold and entered the space that was chosen for her. Each student was given a letter of the alphabet and a message to memorize. As Carrie sat expectantly, each student took turns coming to the microphone to speak a few words that exemplified her character, and then each one proceeded to hand her a long-stemmed red rose.

The first student said, "Carrie, my letter is A, and I want to give you this rose because I think you're amazing." We went through the alphabet until it was time to give out the twenty-sixth rose for the letter Z. The last student said, "Carrie, all of us fourth graders like you and Mr. Z so much that we think it is only fitting if we were to add a Mrs. Zielke, too."

Then it was my turn. If she hadn't gotten it yet, she would soon enough. I stepped up to Carrie from out of the crowd. In an instant, I would learn if I would enter into my time of glory or experience the most embarrassing moment of my life. I was beyond nervous! I fumbled for what felt like an eternity and was finally able to pull the ring out of my pants pocket. I made eye contact with Carrie, got down on one knee, and proposed as she sat on a chair in the center of the dance floor. I was thrilled she said "yes"—I was going to spend the rest of my life with the woman of my dreams.

The future looked extremely bright for us. We couldn't be happier, especially after journeying through cancer together. This extraordinary moment bookmarked a time when I felt alive and rejuvenated, happy to be a man who was living a carefree life.

Reflection Questions

1. Have you had a time when you learned a large number of insights in a short amount of time?

2. How have some of those insights impacted you to this day?

SEEING THE GOOD IN IT

CHAPTER 9

PERSISTENCE, DETERMINATION, AND FEAR OF CONCLUSIONS

Bad memories have a way of haunting a person forever. It could be memories of an inappropriate relationship, an unjust circumstance, or a time when life just threw one punch after another. Whatever the situation, in days, weeks, and years that follow, each of us can find ourselves at familiar and unwelcome intersections that resemble our past. When blindsided by the strong emotions that follow these events, a tsunami of fears threatens to overtake us. We know decisions we make at this time will very likely impact our future and must be made with persistence, determination, and courage. While standing at the precipice, we hear the cacophony we wish to escape. At that dire moment, there's nothing more to do but take a deep breath, think logically, and learn to separate all the clatter to fully understand the next steps that will, hopefully, bring us closer to peace.

For cancer patients, anything closely resembling an ache or pain experienced during your battle against cancer makes you wonder what your future holds. In April 2005, one year after my initial diagnosis, I noticed some slight pain in my hips again. I didn't immediately take it as a serious threat. Sort of like a severe thunderstorm watch, I treated it like a slight annoyance and decided to monitor the situation. I waited a few days to see if the pain would go away or at least lessen.

To my dismay, my hips throbbed more severely with each passing day. My thoughts began to fill with fear. *Make it stop! Please! This cannot be happening.* My future looked so bright, especially with the upcoming marriage to my amazing fiancée on the horizon. I couldn't wait to jump into the American dream of purchasing our first house together. The desire to have a family resurfaced again now that I had a clean bill of health. We felt strongly that we were entering the best days of our lives and that nothing could hold us back after all we'd been through together. I was determined to stay healthy, so if I thought there was the slightest possibility of a recurrence of my cancer, I knew it would be wise to schedule a doctor's visit. Even if all is well, I thought, I would at least have greater peace of mind. So, in the midst of wedding preparations, I decided to call the doctor and let him know I was experiencing some hip pain.

Hearing the doctor verbalize that I still had a clean bill of health would be all I needed to put my worries to rest. As a precaution, my doctor and nurse planned to run a gamut of tests on me. I decided to downplay any upcoming tests, especially for Carrie and my family, because I didn't want to cause anyone undue worry. As I was anticipating the test results, I remember thinking there was no way I could enter this fight again. I barely made it through the first time. If the cancer came back, I wasn't even sure I wanted to put myself through all the trauma of treatment again. I knew from past experience that, sometimes, there is no quality of life during a cancer journey. Thankfully, the tests showed no problem and Carrie, my family, and I welcomed the good news with open arms.

I returned to teaching the very next day with a rejuvenated spirit. However, my hip pains continued to grow more intense, and I had to give myself countless pep talks throughout the day to cope with it. *You're fine, Phil; it's just your imagination.* But deep down inside I knew the pain coming from my bones was sufficient cause for growing concern. I waited a few more days, but could not ignore the escalating intensity of the pain, which was now causing me to lose sleep at night. How could this be happening again? Such hip pain is usually a sign of cancer at its most advanced stage. This was confusing because I didn't have any other symptoms. Besides, a slow-growing cancer couldn't progress to an advanced stage that quickly, could it?

I wanted to put my worries to rest and called the doctor to explain the intensifying problem. He asked me to come back to the hospital for more tests. I decided not to tell Carrie or my mom at this point—it would have worried them beyond comprehension. The only person who knew was my dad.

The doctor scheduled a bone marrow biopsy. There is nothing even remotely fun about getting a needle screwed into your hip bones while awake, then waiting to find out whether or not you're still in remission. Yes, that test was no picnic, but amazingly, it also brought me some laughs that day. You might be thinking to yourself, just how sick and twisted is this guy?

Where is the humor in a situation like that? Let me explain.

Prior to the test, the doctors kindly hinted to my dad to exit the room, but he opted to stay and watch. He videoed my first bone marrow biopsy and he figured he was going to be a tough guy. I supported his decision. However, he probably should have thought twice about this choice. My family has an enduring joke about Dad's very low pain threshold and his apprehension to be in a hospital. This joke has been ongoing since the day I was born, when he passed out after the doctor explained that my mom would need a C-section.

He remained in the room for my bone marrow biopsy, and, true to his character, my dad passed out during the test. The doctor was screwing a long needle into my bone when I suddenly heard a lot of commotion. The doctors had to leave my side to attend to my dad who was about to fall to the floor. I shook my head and laughed out loud as I lay on the operating table watching my medical team attend to this unexpected situation.

Later that day, I again received word from the doctor that the tests showed no sign of cancer. In many cases this would bring amazing relief. Unfortunately, my worries didn't diminish because the intense pain in my hips had not subsided. I knew my body very well at this point, and I could tell without a shadow of a doubt that something was terribly wrong. So, once again, determined to get some answers, I reached out to my doctor and he asked me to come back the following day so they could run one final test.

I didn't sleep well that night. It's not unusual for me to stay up extra late when a critical test is scheduled for the following day. I find it's better to arrive at the hospital exhausted because then I'm less attentive to the details that could trouble me and can relax more easily. Going through the motions half awake has its advantages.

The following morning, I was especially fearful. The possibility that I might have cancer again and what that might mean for Carrie, my family, and me was too terrifying to consider. The seriousness of the circumstances hit me in the face when I arrived in the operating room. The medical team preparing to work on me was twice the size used the day before. Besides, this was a test I'd never had before, so I didn't know what to expect. To make matters worse, I was told that the procedure was called a CT-guided needle biopsy. I wasn't looking forward to any part of that.

The plan was to screw an eight-inch hollow needle into my hip bone while I was awake. The CT scans would be repeated until they could guide the needle into the suspicious area to get a sample. I would rather have been anywhere else in that moment. It took all the strength of more than a few people to precisely screw the needle in and a few more to hold me down as I grimaced in pain. I gripped the towel in front of me with all my might, as if I was hanging on to a cliff for dear life.

The test was unbearable. After each CT scan, they moved the needle a little more through my hip bone until they were finally in the right location. Once they navigated the needle to its destination, they inserted another needle inside the hollow needle to extract fluid for the biopsy. I prayed more earnestly and desperately than I had ever prayed before in my life. I clenched my fists and let out more than a few grunts as I bit down on the towel in front of me.

My broken body hurt so much after this excruciating test that I walked with a limp for the next few days. I had never felt more violated in my life. "Can I have some more pain medication, please?" was my recurring plea. To make matters worse, I had to endure the time it took for the pathologist to analyze the test results. I didn't know what news was looming around the corner, but I did cognitively understand it could possibly alter my life in unimaginable ways. I had an inkling that my doctor had already suspected what was coming, and I was about to find out soon enough.

***

When the direction in our life hits an abrupt turning point, we can experience intense emotions that can alter our ability to make wise, logical decisions. The heaviness of fear bears down on us, making it difficult to find the strength and courage we need to move forward. At any time when fear intersects with our ability to make clear, informed decisions, it becomes important to proceed carefully, balancing caution and persistence. Standing in one place for a long period of time causes us to grow tired and weary, and at some point, we will discover it no longer will be a sustainable option for us. But, as time goes on, an epiphany can take hold as we discover the importance of staying the course to see what awaits us on the other side.

Reflection Questions

1. What have setbacks looked like for you in your suffering? Have you ever had to advocate for yourself when you know something is wrong but others don't agree?

2. How do you make decisions well when intense emotions over whelm you?

CHAPTER 10

THE PROMISE OF RAINBOWS

⌘

When we make promises, we're giving affirmation for the future. We show our intention when we use words and phrases such as "I swear," "I vow," "I guarantee," "I pledge," or "I give you my word." A promise kept creates harmony and peace in any union—which is a necessary foundation for all healthy relationships. A broken promise, in contrast, can break trust. But, in some situations, it's not possible for a person to make a promise because they're not sure it's one they can keep.

When it comes to our health, doctors can't make any promises. Typically we go to the doctor for routine maintenance or to figure out what's gone so terribly wrong. We undergo various forms of medical procedures with the intention that we'll soon be given an explanation. We're given the assurance that they will get to the bottom of it. If the doctor reports to us all is well, we can once again relax and breathe easier. However, if the news shows ill health or an occurrence of cancer, the only thing we're promised is a challenging journey ahead. Doctors can give us statistics on survival rates or possible side effects from the treatment, but they cannot promise the outcome. Thankfully, there are some promises available that bring an everlasting hope to all of us, no matter what situation we find ourselves facing.

***

I was at home in my bedroom when I received the long-awaited news. The doctor called a few short hours after my test and his update instantly took my breath away. The biopsy results showed a couple of cancer cells that were still active. "There must have been a cell hiding somewhere," he said. My life and my future flashed before me. The cancer was still stage 4B, and with the new diagnosis, death was an even greater possibility. The news grew progressively worse the deeper into the conversation we went. I felt as if my life, my dreams, and my future were deflating fast, and all I could do was stand there and watch it happen.

Regret set in as the doctor informed me that, in hindsight, he wished they had done things differently the first time around. "If we could turn back the clock, we wouldn't have stopped treatment so soon," he reflected. He said they should have continued with a stem cell transplant and radiation afterward, explaining that the chemotherapy treatment repressed the cancer so much it was undetectable on the scans. This time around, they decided to attack the cancer ten times more aggressively for a hundred times the effect. They needed a few days to determine the best course of action, so he suggested I take the weekend to gather myself, pack a bag, and come back to the hospital on Monday for an extended stay. How was I supposed to respond to this devastating news? "Thanks for calling and have a good day"? I can't recall what else we said during the remainder of the conversation, but it didn't matter anyway.

I buried my face in my hands as my emotions swept over me. Furious protests rose from the depths of my soul and exploded outside the surface of my control. Anger and resentment didn't enter my thoughts the first time I was diagnosed because, after being sick for so long, I was just happy they could do something about it. This time around, it couldn't have been more different. I was mad at God, and I was mad at the world. I simply didn't understand why this was happening to me. My greatest fear was upon me, and nobody could shake me hard enough to wake me from this nightmare.

I was unsure how I wanted to proceed. Should I take my own life to avoid all the stress and pain? Should I decline treatment until cancer could bring my life to an end? If I agreed to treatment, there would be no guarantee it would work anyway. What would my quality of life look like if I accepted treatment? Did I have to throw my dream of living a peaceful life away once again?

Was this really happening?

After digesting all the incomprehensible information, the scariest part for me wasn't hearing the news, but sharing it with those I loved. I dreaded the intense pain this was going to cause the people who cared so deeply for me. How would I tell my fiancée there might not be a wedding after all and that she might never have me as her husband? *God, help me! This news will crush her.* This was truly a moment of hysteria.

Once I gathered my thoughts as much as humanly possible, I knew there was only one course of action to take: fight cancer again! Quitting was not a part of my DNA. And this time I wasn't just fighting for myself. I was fighting for my fiancée and for my family.

My dad and I had a heart-to-heart about the action steps that needed to take place regarding who to tell and in what order. Talking with him gave me clarity. Carrie needed to know first. She was planning to come over to my parents' house after work anyway, so I would wait until then. I asked my dad not to share the news with anyone else, not even my mom—not yet. I didn't want her to worry and stress out any sooner than necessary.

The next day was going to have to be the final day with my fourth-grade students. My principal needed to know how to proceed as soon as possible so he could find a replacement for me until the end of the school year. My dad and I drove to the school. My principal took the news as well as could be expected and helped me figure out when and how to share the news with the faculty and, most importantly, with the nine- and ten-year-olds in my class. We decided that I would craft an email to my colleagues that night to send out in the morning. On my list for the next day was to share the news with my fourth graders. This wasn't going to be an easy task. But nothing in the near future was going to be easy.

By the time I got home that day, I was exhausted and emotionally drained. I sat alone in silence in the front room, waiting for Carrie to pull into the driveway. My desire to see her was unwavering, but I dreaded the moment when I had to tell her the news. It would, without a doubt, shatter her world. I tried to prepare myself for this unbearable moment, rehearsing the words and her reaction over and over in my mind. Finally, whether I was ready or not, she arrived.

I opened the car door and managed a welcoming smile. We embraced and I gave her a kiss that told her how much she meant to me. I held her hand as we walked toward the backyard. We stopped on the driveway, she turned toward me, and we locked eyes. "I talked to the doctor today and he gave me the test results." Her face instantly showed her apprehension. I took a deep breath and said the words nobody ever wants to hear themselves say: "I have cancer." She started crying instantly. She shook her head, denying the news. I held her tight as she fell into my arms and sobbed. I absorbed all her body weight as she cried like I had never seen her cry before. I couldn't do anything except hold her and do my best to console her, but I knew nothing I could say at that moment would help. I couldn't tell her everything was OK because it wasn't. And I wasn't sure it ever would be. It felt like my heart and feelings were a million miles away from my mind while I simultaneously hated seeing her in so much pain. Time was standing still. I had just delivered news to the girl I loved that we would have to postpone our wedding. In fact, I'd told the woman of my dreams there might never be a wedding. Reality had set in: Carrie knew now that she might lose me altogether. This shook both of us to the core, more than anything in our lives had ever done. We had already journeyed through so much together, but this was a new challenge we didn't know we'd ever get through.

Later that night we sat in the kitchen as a family while I prepared to tell my mom, brother, and sisters the awful news. My mom had asked my dad earlier in the day if we had received the test results, and he followed through with my wishes not to tell anyone yet. But I couldn't put it off any longer. The dreaded announcement brought more shock and tears. I remained stoic as I watched each family member grapple with the news in their own way. I couldn't console them, and I didn't bother trying. All I could do was be as stable as possible, which didn't seem doable to me at all. We knew the devastation that cancer had caused us only a year earlier. The second time was much worse for all of us because we knew what was coming—pain, trauma, and many more trials, with no guarantees about the future. Once it was clear that there was no more to say, I left the room. I certainly didn't want to be part of a pity party. Maybe it was my way of avoiding and ignoring the pain altogether. Sometimes that's all we can do.

I had trouble sleeping that night, and I'm sure that was the case for my family as well. The next day I awoke to the same nightmare staring me in the face. My hips were throbbing more intensely with every waking hour. Early that morning I sent the email with the news to the faculty and staff at the school. Various individuals came to my classroom throughout the day to share a few heartfelt words and to let me know I was in their thoughts and prayers. There was no need or desire for any extended conversations. I was just trying to make it through the day.

As a teacher, I had made hundreds of lesson plans, and each year I became better at planning due to my prior teaching experiences. However, no previous experience prepared me for what took place later that day when I had to share the update with my students. Whether it was working on math facts or doing hands-on science experiments, I loved being with those kids. Teaching isn't for the faint of heart and the days weren't always easy, but they were always worth it. Throughout the day, memories from the school year cycled through my mind. I would deeply miss each and every student in my class.

An hour before school would close for the day, I led my students outside in a single file line. It was a bright, sunny day, and I had informed the class earlier that if we went above and beyond, the day would end with a special recess. They always responded positively to such a challenge. When the time came, we ventured outside to the playground for a class meeting and the extra recess. The solemn news I had to share weighed heavily on me. Thankfully everything had gone according to plan and word did not get out, so none of the students had a clue as to what I was about to say.

We opened the class meeting with informal chatting and then it was time to share. I told the students, "I have been undergoing tests for cancer again, and yesterday I received some news I didn't want to hear. The cancer has returned. I'm even sorrier to say that this is going to be my last day to teach you this year." As I looked around the circle at the expressions of these nine-and ten-year-olds, I saw worried and sad faces looking back at me. One student started crying, and before I knew it, the tears had spread to everyone around the circle.

Teaching in a parochial setting allowed me to share my personal faith with my students on a daily basis. At no other time was I more thankful to be given the opportunity to be so honest about the thoughts and emotions that were flooding my mind. I didn't want to lose a teachable moment and a chance to comfort my students, so I started talking about God's promises. I made eye contact with each of them as I reminded them how God had taken care of me the first time I had cancer, and he would take care of me again. We talked about Noah and how God used the ark to save Noah's family and the animals. Tears started welling up in my eyes as I spoke. My class needed to hear this message of good news, but my heart desperately needed to hear it as well. I continued this impromptu lesson by asking my class, "What was the sign that God sent Noah to remind him and everyone that he is always with us and will never send a flood to destroy the Earth again?" One student raised his hand and said, "Mr. Z, he sent a rainbow." Before I could even respond, I looked up in the sky and nearly lost it as tears streamed down my face. I couldn't believe what I saw. At that very moment, in the expansive sky above us, was the most beautiful rainbow I'd ever seen. I was speechless. Tears of pain and tears of joy flooded my face. God's promise was once again showing up in a way I had least expected. What an emotional way to end the day!

***

We are all well aware that living in the world doesn't guarantee any of us a life free from trouble. Bodies break down, people disappoint us, and our plans don't always go as expected. Nobody leaves this world unscathed. At rock bottom, we begin to understand that hope cannot be found solely by trusting in ourselves or others for our victory. Fears of abandonment can take over, leaving us with a feeling of despair. But, even in our troubled world, the sight of a spectacular rainbow in an outstretched sky can become a welcome sign reminding us that, in sickness and in health, God's promise never fails—and it is a guaranteed gift that will stand the test of time.

Reflection Questions

1. What promises of God do you cling to when life otherwise feels hopeless?

2. Think of a time when God showed up for you a way you least expected it, reminding you that he is always with you.

SEEING THE GOOD IN IT

CHAPTER 11

I NEED A LIFELINE, PLEASE

◈

Have you ever had one of those days that is so bad you think it will never end? In the heat of the moment, without speaking a single word, we send warning signals to everyone around us with our frustrated energy. Our blood pressure rises, the vein in our forehead begins to pulsate, and before we know it, our jaw clenches and we can't think clearly.

***

When you're in the middle of cancer treatment, it seems as though everything that can go wrong does go wrong. The beast becomes your reality and overwhelms you. The dynamic duo—complications and stress—increase the intensity and become too much to handle. You feel like you're barely hanging on in such times of desperation. Worst of all, your spirit is crushed while your body is failing.

I was trying to hold on with all my might. The weekend was over, and I found myself back at the hospital, once again engaging in a fight for life. It was as if the doctor put a mask on and turned into an evil game show host. "Congratulations, Phil, you pulled the lucky number. Come on down, and let's show everyone what you've won. You've won a once-in-a-lifetime opportunity to battle cancer for the second time. Wait, there's more! The treatment you'll be given will be ten times more aggressive than the first time you had cancer and will be—don't miss this, everyone—one hundred times tougher on your body and emotions. Your regimen will consist of six cycles of chemotherapy, a stem cell transplant, AND radiation. Now, Phil, it's time to head off to surgery to place a port in your chest. Only this time it will be more of a struggle as we reopen old wounds and work through built-up scar tissue. Let's all congratulate him on what he's won." Is that a bit silly and overstated? Sure, but I'm confident that anyone who has battled cancer can relate. I told myself, *It's time to buckle down for the duration. Everything this time around is going to take longer. The treatment will be much more aggressive, and the stakes will be much higher. Win, lose, or draw, this is my lot, and I can't do anything about it.* Can you sense the frustration I felt?

Only three days into chemotherapy, I was already confined to my hospital bed and feeling worse than I did after any previous treatment. I became sick within hours of starting the new regimen, and the antinausea and pain medication couldn't keep up. Complications were recurring and appearing at unexpected times. Frustration, anger, and resentment took over. When strong emotions are kept at bay for long periods of time, they eventually have to surface somewhere in some way.

For the next three days, I laid in my hospital bed becoming more distraught with each passing moment until I finally reached my boiling point. On top of the cancer itself, my state of mind was also harming me. I was so angry and upset that I considered getting out of bed and running directly into the hospital wall in front of me in hopes of breaking through it. I was fuming and extremely unstable. *Watch out, everyone; stay out of my way! You don't have to tick me off—I'm already ticked off! It doesn't matter what you say or do or what your intentions are,*

I will find a way to make you suffer! Don't even look at me wrong! Rage was spilling out of me in every way possible, and it wasn't just because of the physical parts of the cancer. I was wrestling with the fact that my entire future may have just been stolen from me.

One night at three in the morning, I was so unsettled I couldn't sleep. It was no surprise that my blood pressure and heart rate were off the charts. My dad was sleeping on the couch in my hospital room as he did most nights. He woke up to my hysterical screaming and pleading with God at the top of my lungs: "God, how could you let this happen?! Why did you have to take everything away from me again?! Didn't I learn what you wanted me to learn the first time around? My fourth graders are suffering too! I thought I was making a difference in their lives and for your kingdom. Didn't you see that? Why?!" I started sobbing and streams of tears made their way down my face. I could barely get the words out. "What about Carrie? Not only am I crushed, but you've crushed her too! How could you do this to us? All my plans and all my dreams are gone!"

In that moment, I was a child that couldn't be calmed down or consoled. Nothing that could have been said at that time would have comforted me. I needed to wrestle with the reality of the situation. I continued to pour my heart out to God. Eventually I ran out of steam and the hysteria diminished. The sobbing slowed down, and the room became silent again, except for the incessant *beep, beep, beep* that came from the medical devices that seemed to be forever a part of me.

I was so worn out by the trauma and stress of the past few days that I started to fall asleep from sheer exhaustion. When I finally did close my weary eyes, it was as if I heard a clear whisper from God. *"Are you ready to stop fighting this with your own strength? You will keep struggling like this if you continue to try to do it all on your own. Why don't you give the cancer to me so I can fight this battle for you?"* In that moment, it hit me—I didn't need to feel alone in my battle if I didn't want to. The ultimate reason I was struggling so much with the recurrence of my cancer was because I was trying to fight it on my own. I finally realized that it was time for me to give the situation completely over to God. He became my lifeline. Once I turned it over to him, I didn't feel as though I needed to be the one in control. Once I made the decision to take it out of my hands and put it in his, a complete sense of peace swept over me. I knew this sense of peace would be hard to sustain with everything coming at me at such a fast clip. But no matter what came my way, whether I felt the peace in that moment or not, I grew to understand that God was my lifeline who wanted me to desperately reach out, grab hold of his hand, and discover that peace once again.

The next day, my reliance on God was put to the test. I woke up in much worse shape, and I felt like I was literally dying. But Carrie and my brother Joel were graduating from college that day. I didn't care how much trauma I felt—I wanted to be there no matter what. I had already missed so much, and I didn't want to have any regrets about this day. Even though I was as sick as I had ever been in my life, I begged my doctor to let me return home from the hospital. He knew I was trying my best to make it to the graduation that day and allowed me to go home.

My parents planned to hold a graduation party at our house after the ceremony. Family and friends were going to gather in droves from long distances to celebrate. In spite of my determination to attend the graduation and celebrate with my family at the party, I soon realized my intentions and determination weren't enough. Throughout the afternoon, I could only move back and forth from my bed to the toilet to throw up every few minutes. Reality hit that I was not going to make it to the ceremony.

Nausea was a common experience for me while I was undergoing chemotherapy. Any smell could set it off—it was like a ticking time bomb, and the various food smells in the house weren't helping the situation. When everyone arrived for the party, I began to smell the barbecue beef that was cooking in the crockpot circulating through the air vents into my bedroom. Previously this had been one of my favorite smells, but one whiff set off an unprecedented amount of nausea. I had nothing left to throw up, but I couldn't make it stop.

I struggled down the stairs through a crowd of people, hoping nobody would notice me. I needed to get out! I made my way out the front door, lowering my head as I tried to keep from passing out. The fresh air was beckoning me. The last thing I wanted to do was see people, but I had to go through the crowd to get outside. When I finally got outside, I asked a friend to get my dad so that he could take me back to the hospital. We got to the hospital in record time. It's a miracle the police didn't pull us over. When we got there, I opened the car door as quickly as I could and immediately fell face down in the grass outside the emergency room. The short few hours outside the hospital had been too much for me to handle. I would be in the hospital for the next three weeks. The rest of the world went on with their lives, going from destination A to destination B, while I was stuck in one place, staring at a wall that never changed. You miss out on a lot when you're going through cancer, and at times, you feel forgotten. My single greatest desire was to be set free from this torture chamber.

***

When we find ourselves stuck in a cycle of bad days, when life hits us with one sucker punch after another, it seems as though we can't help ourselves and nobody else can help either. It's as if we're shoved into an elevator against our will and the doors have closed tightly behind us. No matter how much we scream, there's nobody there to hear our plea for help. Isolated, we begin to panic. With no way out, we fall to our knees and weep. Reality sinks in that we're stuck in this dark, secluded, godforsaken place that is not meant to be our permanent residence. Once we're there, two choices remain: stay in the depths of despair or pray to the God of the universe that he will come to our rescue. For some, reaching out may be a new experience. For others, it's a comforting reminder and a reassurance that we are not alone, something for which to be thankful. No matter what, calling out to the Almighty will provide a sense of peace, allowing the chasm between you and God to slowly diminish. Having nothing to lose, we throw our hands into the air in total desperation and hurl a prayer toward Heaven to let God know we are lost.

When we draw near to God, our vantage point begins to change as we come to realize we are not alone. He meets us throughout the day—on our hospital bed, at home, in the car, or when we feel like we're trapped in a dark elevator. When we tell him we're sad, upset, ashamed, or regretful, he mysteriously meets us in the midst of it all. As we spend quiet time meditating on God's promises, it becomes easier to feel the undeniable peace that washes over us and the depth of his everlasting love that is freely given. Finally, to get through the unpredictable circumstances that life throws our way, we come to realize God truly is our only viable option.

Reflection Questions

1. Have you ever reached a moment when you realized you could no longer fight with your own strength?

2. When you're in the depths of despair, how do you cry out to God?

CHAPTER 12

TRANSPLANT DAY

❧

Gardening is a precise task. Plants need appropriate spacing in rich soil, beams of sunlight, and water to survive. If even one element is missing, chances of survival are slim, and it may be that the only option left is to try to transplant it to a new location. Transplants are risky, but if nothing is done, death is certain. In such cases, gardeners carefully begin the process and execute a plan. The most fragile time in the life of that dying plant is during and immediately after the transplant takes place. And even executed with the most careful preparation and painstaking care, gardeners understand that the transplant still may not be successful.

Due to the miracle of modern medicine, people can get transplants as well. When a doctor tells us a transplant is our only chance for survival, the news sends welding-sized sparks of emotions flying in every direction and makes us acutely aware that our expiration date is approaching. Even if we do qualify after testing, and they move forward with the procedure, we're informed that more risky challenges will most likely follow. Although the likelihood of receiving a transplant is higher today than in the past, many individuals still lose the fight because the timing never lines up, other organs might have failed in the process, or their body rejects it.

My six months of treatment continued into July, and everyone knew the next part would be the riskiest yet. My body was worn down, and in that depleted state, I had to prep for a procedure that could very well end my life: a stem cell transplant. It was going to be a miracle if I made it through to the other side.

To prepare for the transplant procedure, I underwent minor surgery to place an in-and-out tube into my neck. Next, they harvested my stem cells (similar to dialysis). The blood circulated in and out of my body through the tubes for two days, and the medical team collected some of my stem cells in a bag. Finally, the cells were frozen until it was time for the transplant. Fortunately, I was able to use my own stem cells. This was the best-case scenario because it would be extremely unlikely for my body to reject my own blood. When it was finally over, the whole experience left me light-headed with a pounding headache and nausea.

After that grueling experience, the doctors sent me home to "rest" for a few days. When I returned to the hospital I received seven days of lethal chemotherapy. My blood count plummeted. If these numbers fell any further, I was told with certainty that I wouldn't make it past the next day. The interminable oxygen mask helped me to breathe, and the assorted tubes pumped in the required nutrients. On the brink of death, as I lay in my isolation room getting ready for my stem cell transplant, I was in unbearable pain and wondered if I would live to see the next day.

I looked toward the door and saw a large group of people that I didn't recognize congregating outside. At this point I wasn't sure what was happening. Were all these people here because something had gone terribly wrong? As soon as that thought crept into my mind, a few people dressed in white from head to toe entered my room. I didn't move at all other than to turn my eyes toward them. Everything is different when your blood counts are low and you're at the point of death. It was as though I was having an out-of-body experience. I was there, but I wasn't fully present. The nurse stated, "Phil, it's Kelly. It's transplant day." I knew Kelly well; she was my nurse practitioner. They hooked up the IV to my port and all the stem cells drained into my body.

Hallucinations, tremors, and excruciating pain made seconds feel like minutes and minutes feel like hours. It seemed as if time was standing still. Merely hoping for the best didn't change my circumstances.

After the procedure, as I looked into the mirror in front of me, all I saw was a worn-out face with no eyelashes, shriveled-up veins, and weakened bones underneath my paper-thin skin. My body's complexion had turned from white to a shade of gray. The sores inside my mouth and up and down my esophagus were unbearable, making drinking even a sip of water nearly impossible. For the next few weeks, I received much needed morphine around the clock, but nothing seemed to provide relief.

One day I glanced at the whiteboard in my room, which listed the date: August 13, 2005. Although I was in excruciating pain, I remembered that two of my good friends, Jen and Ryan, were getting married that day. The cancer that I wore daily should have been a reminder that I would not be able to attend this special event. However, that day I woke up from my nap with a sense of urgency, worried about being late to the wedding. In my disorientated state of mind, I thought I could leave the hospital and join the festivities. I looked around the room. To my surprise, no one was there to help me. *That's odd*, I thought. But I proceeded to get ready by myself. Even though I was obviously too ill and under the influence of a lot of heavy-duty drugs, I was determined to be part of this special day. So I disconnected my IV pole, took off the oxygen mask, removed the IVs from my arms, and detached the needle from the port in my chest. I inched my way to the edge of the bed to put on my sweat jacket over my bare skin, and then proceeded to leave the room with the energy and feeble movement of a ninety-year-old man. I only retreated a few steps into the hallway when the nurses noticed me heading toward the exit.

They wouldn't let me leave, and I couldn't fathom why. Didn't they know it's rude to be late to a wedding? About the time that thought crossed my mind, I looked down and saw blood dripping at a slow and steady pace below my chest, over my exposed arms, and against my white shorts. The blood, now flowing like a lazy river, gradually splattered onto the clean, tiled floor.

The bleeding should have been enough to convince me that I was in no shape to attend a wedding, but my confused brain ignored the message. I was determined to make it to the next important date on my calendar. I didn't want to miss out on the party. I finally came to my senses and was escorted safely back to my awaiting bed.

Throughout the day, I pressed the red button for relief as often as I could. I continually felt like I needed more morphine to ease the perpetual pain. *Why are these drugs not doing their job? I'll page the nurse and demand stronger pain medication.* The nurses explained to me that there was nothing else they could give me. They couldn't give me any more than the doctor ordered. There was no way this response was good enough for me. So, without hesitation, I demanded, "Page the doctor, NOW!"

The attending doctor and his colleagues arrived and explained that I'd been given all the medication allowed. Again, the answer didn't satisfy me—the physician obviously needed to provide me with a better explanation. "Don't you know how I feel?" I yelled out. I mustered up enough energy to argue with the doctor in an attempt to get what I wanted. However, my argument didn't convince him. I had already consumed all the drugs my body could tolerate. My life was enveloped in a heavy cloud. Chemo brain set in as the storm within and around me grew with intensity. Having a conversation was a lost cause. The two big wires that were supposed to connect in my brain to complete a thought had been severed and were flying around out of control. It was obvious that the drugs brought the worst out in me and I was quickly losing touch with reality. In this condition, it was hard for me to see outside my circumstances, and I knew that it was definitely difficult for others to see within.

***

We all have wounds that affect our ability to survive. In the case of a dying plant, a transplant may be the only option for survival. With a little help from nature and a capable gardener to carry out the necessary plans, chances are that the plant may survive. In the same way, when we get a green light for transplant, the doctors inform us that they will develop a comprehensive action plan with the intention of moving forward with precision to save our life. We understand the high risks associated with transplants, but we also know that if we choose not to move ahead the only option available to us will be death.

There are many miracles in modern medicine, yet an even greater miracle is that our bodies were created to rejuvenate. It's no coincidence that our ultimate desire when sick is to return to our original form. Our strong yearning to be healthy reminds us that God's intentional design for our bodies is perfect. Therefore, no matter what problems we face today or even tomorrow, we can be confident and have great joy in knowing that these challenges won't remain with us throughout eternity.

Reflection Questions

1. What hope does it give you to know that our bodies will be perfect in eternity?

2. What gift of the modern world can you thank God for because of the way it has helped you, despite living in a broken world?

TRANSPLANT DAY

CHAPTER 13

CHANGING FROM THE INSIDE OUT

You've probably heard the profound statement, "In the end, it's not the years in your life that count; it's the life in your years." So how do we experience more life in our years? Abraham Lincoln encourages us with his sage advice: "Leave nothing for tomorrow which can be accomplished today." In other words, be mindful of the opportunities that life brings us today to make a difference in our life tomorrow. A cross country runner who wants to stay with the lead pack decides to train a little more each day. A public speaker who wants to be more engaging delivers a talk to multiple audiences and tweaks his presentation along the way. A parent who hopes their relationship with their child will grow is deliberate about spending time together.

Change may feel borderline impossible, yet lasting change is necessary for a life well lived. As we lie in our hospital bed or sit in our chair, we may wonder, *Where will I be in six months? What will I feel like? How will I be different than I am today?* Taking on small improvements one day at a time catapults us into a different stratosphere. However, it's easier said than done when our body is compromised and vulnerable to attack from the inside out.

***

Three weeks after my stem cell transplant, I couldn't tolerate being in the hospital one second longer. I felt like I was going crazy. My blood counts were starting to rise to normal levels, but I still needed around-the-clock medical care. However, if I didn't get a change of scenery, I didn't think I was going to emotionally survive. I knew that staying positive and maintaining good emotional health was crucial to my healing process. Once I lost my will to fight, the chances of making it through the transplant procedure were going to be reduced considerably. Without a change in scenery, I could sense I was on the edge of giving up.

I needed to get my point across to the doctor, but thinking and talking were two of the many things I didn't have enough energy to do. It hurt to think and it hurt to talk. I only spoke when something was literally a matter of life or death. I could barely open my eyes and had not spoken more than a few words in weeks. Mostly I just nodded my head.

One day, I conserved my energy so I could talk with the doctor. When the time came, it took all my strength to whisper a few words. I told him that if I didn't get out of this prison, I didn't think I was going to make it. He shared with me that they had never let anyone go home this early in the history of doing stem cell transplants. I pleaded with him to let me leave. He checked me over and told me he would be back in a few minutes.

When he came back, he told me, "Phil, I will let you go home. However, you will need to go home on an IV, and we will set up home medical care for you. I need to see you back here at the hospital tomorrow morning so we can monitor you closely and each day thereafter. As long as you're progressing according to plan, after a period of time, you won't need to come in every day. As always, you can call me day or night. Got it, Star?" (Star was his nickname for me). I opened my eyes and nodded my head the slightest bit.

A few of my nurses entered a short time later dumbfounded and visibly upset. You could tell they had just wiped tears from their eyes. They strongly encouraged me not to go. This was their last-ditch effort to keep me in the hospital, but nothing was going to change how firmly I felt about my exit plan. "The doctor said I can go," I responded. My nurses were like family to me. They knew the severity of the situation, and they wanted what was best for me. My doctor wanted what was best for me as well, but he was a bit more lenient, and we all knew it. I'm glad he was. I loved each of them and greatly appreciated their caring for me.

My body was shaking a lot at this point (as it often did), but I managed to sit on the edge of my bed and reach for the phone to call Carrie. "Come get me. I'm going home," I told her. She paused, and then responded with skepticism, "Really?" I replied with a simple "Yes." Then the nausea set in. I set the phone on the bed for a moment and attempted to walk to the bathroom, but it was too late. I couldn't say much more because my body suddenly reacted in violent, messy ways. "Phil, are you OK? Are you OK?" After a minute or so, I was able to gather myself to answer her, "Call my dad and come get me." We ended our conversation with that final request. Everyone close to me was in a state of disbelief. They thought going home was a bad idea, but I couldn't stand being in the hospital any longer. No one could force me to stay. It may sound crazy, but at that moment, I was sure my life depended on getting home to my own bed.

A few hours later, Carrie and my dad arrived at the hospital. It was going to be some time before all the paperwork was processed, so we started the routine that had come naturally to us while waiting. My dad always liked to have food sent up to the room from the cafeteria. It used to secretly aggravate me when he ordered food because I couldn't eat at all, and the smell would make me nauseous. However, I never voiced my opinion because he sacrificed so much for me. I'd just roll my eyes every time he ordered.

Carrie decided to place the order this time. She went to the phone, dialed, and put the receiver up to her ear. I watched as a look of disgust came over her face and she cried out, "Oh, man, what's all over the phone?" I was able to put two and two together and quickly determine what the disgusting substance was. Carrie and my dad figured it out too. Instantly, we all busted up laughing. I hadn't even cracked a smile in weeks. It was funny to me, and secretly I felt like I had gained a little revenge for all the times he'd eaten food in front of me in my hospital room. But I did feel bad about what had happened for another reason—I knew the nurse would have to clean up the mess. When I paged for help, I was greeted by a new nurse in her early twenties. This was not only the first time she took care of me—it was her first day on the job. *I'm really sorry about the mess and, by the way, welcome to nursing.*

Over the course of the afternoon, the nurses came in, changed my bandages, and finally disconnected me from the IV pole. The IVs would still be active, but now instead of dragging the IV pole behind me, as I was accustomed to doing, I carried a backpack. I felt as if I was bringing the entire pharmacy with me so I could continue with all the medications I needed. As one of my nurses wheeled me onto the elevator, she started crying. It was an emotional time for her after being through so much with me. I was thankful for all the support she and others had given me, but even more thankful to get out of the hospital.

The last few weeks stuck inside the hospital had been a blur, and I still didn't see an end in sight. Now I was scheduled to return to the hospital every day until further notice. I received blood transfusions on and off for the next few weeks, and each transfusion brought some form of relief. With time, the sores in my throat and esophagus had begun to heal, so I started drinking water again. My blood counts began to rise, and in early September, I was given the go ahead to have medical care come home to me.

Toward the end of September, I started to have some more normal living experiences. I began to eat solid foods again. However, I wasn't prepared for the aftermath of that daily ritual. When you start eating solid foods after a few months without doing so, you encounter more pain. For the next month, I dreaded using the restroom. I had taken a lot of things for granted prior to cancer, and relearning some of them was painful and difficult.

That ninth month of that year was a month I wanted to forget altogether. Devastation from my storm was all around me and threatened to consume me. I realize now that a lot had happened in one month, and through it all, there was no denying that I was changing slowly but surely from the inside out. A song by Green Day continually ran through my head: "Summer has come and passed, the innocent can never last. Wake me up when September ends." Even today when hearing that song, I'm brought back to that dark month when I was caught in the middle of my own unrelenting battle and couldn't wait for September to end.

Reflection Questions

1. How can you celebrate the small improvements in the midst of your suffering?

2. What changes can you make to improve your mental state, even if your circumstances don't change?

CHAPTER 14

NEEDING AN ATTITUDE ADJUSTMENT

❧

Maya Angelou is often quoted as saying, "If you don't like something, change it. If you can't change it, change your attitude." One constant a person faces on their cancer journey is the notion of inevitable change, and sadly, we can do nothing to prevent much of the change that occurs around us. Some of the changes are good, but most are painful, frustrating, and even traumatizing.

Over time, I discovered that not keeping the big picture in mind could slow down my healing process. This sudden revelation showed me I needed to take a step back and look at the journey through a much wider lens. Indeed, this new realization made the process more manageable and victory more attainable.

As I was learning to see the bigger picture, I was also reminded to take stock of the silver linings of the journey. I was extremely grateful to have good friends who would check my emotional pulse to determine how and when to encourage me, which reminded me that my life truly mattered. Whenever I felt worthless, it was easy to lose hope and eventually lose the will to fight. Knowing I was seen and heard restored a sense of dignity within me.

On the toughest days, Carrie would ask me to tell her three things for which I was thankful. Sometimes it was impossible to think of three things. I became extremely frustrated with her for even asking such a question. I would think to myself, *Some nerve she has to ask me a question like that!* Of course, she knew my response meant I'd completely lost my perspective and a lack of hope was taking over. It was during moments like these that I needed a reminder to recalibrate and consider the idea of being thankful.

I had to dig deep to find something worth celebrating, but once I did, a renewed sense of victory followed. For instance, on high pain days when I couldn't do more than lie quietly in my bed, I was grateful to have pain medication. When the pain medication didn't do its job, I was thankful for the knowledge from prior experience that the pain wouldn't last forever. When medical bills looked like a tsunami, I was thankful for all the expenses I'd avoided by having insurance. When I was confined to my bed, I was thankful I had a bed to sleep in. When treatments put me back in the hospital for another unwanted stay, I was thankful I had a place to go and receive around-the-clock advanced medical care. When my body wouldn't recover on its own, I was thankful that people donated blood so that I could live.

A positive attitude fostered greater peace of mind and contributed to my recovery. I knew that choosing to be thankful, no matter the circumstances, kept me moving in the right direction. When I found myself getting off track, thankfully, I had caring people encouraging me and cheering me on to the path of victory. How grateful I was to have discovered that having a thankful heart was important and celebrating each victory, no matter how small, would keep me in the fight.

As time passed, I continued to exercise my right to have a positive attitude. I tried to identify something I could celebrate each day. Soon it became a way of life. I celebrated graduating from sleeping on the couch to moving into my bedroom. Before long I made my way into the kitchen and celebrated by eating whatever appealed to me at the time. Shortly thereafter, when I wasn't totally exhausted, I celebrated by taking a slow walk, even if it was just down to the corner of my block and back. I had an elevated awareness that life is too short not to enjoy it when you can.

The nausea was still constant, but not as strong as it was immediately following the transplant. I still had my travel backpack with my IV attached, but I felt so much freedom. I had been released from taking the day-to-day trek back to the hospital. The nurse came to my home to give me my daily shots and check my blood counts. Thankfully, my counts continued to rise each day.

Around this time, I finally felt up to reading a little bit. Since I had kept a journal the entire time I'd had cancer, I thought it would be a good idea to take out this daily account of my experiences and try to read a few pages. I found the royal blue three-ring binder that was never far from me during my battle with cancer. As I opened this warehouse of memories, I noticed how the cardboard inside the cover was now a little flimsy. Every loose leaf paper was recorded the same— always written in ink with the date in the upper right-hand corner to document each moment in time.

I turned to page one and tried to recall why I began writing in the first place. It all started when my friend and mentor Ruth, who was in her nineties, called me when she heard I had cancer. She didn't waste any time and headed right to the point. "Phil, it's Ruth. I heard you had cancer. I'm sorry. You are going to want to keep a journal and write down what God has done in your life so that you can share your story with the world. I'll be praying for you." Click.

I was so thankful that Ruth suggested I keep a record of my daily fight with cancer. The right words of encouragement spoken at the right time can be profound. Ruth called because she cared deeply for me, and because of her, I can now look back on everything I've been through and call to mind how God, faithfully, brought me through it. As I continued to reflect, I thought about why it was so meaningful to me that this advice came from her. Ruth lived on the corner of our street when I was growing up and she gave me my first job mowing her lawn at the age of eight. Not only would she pay me $20 every time I mowed her lawn, which was a lot back in 1989, but what Ruth said and did after I mowed her lawn was what made a lasting mark on me. The ritual was always the same. When I was finished with my job, I would enter her breezeway. The heavy screen door would slam behind me, and I would take off my grass-stained shoes and place them next to the concrete steps leading up to the weathered, white farm door. Shortly thereafter, I would hear her shuffle her way to the door, unlock the latch, and open the top half so I could see her. She would greet me with a thankful smile and unlock the bottom of the heavy door. I would enter the kitchen and she would slowly walk over to the counter to retrieve her purse. From the corner of my eye I could see the small, emerald-green, circular cookie tin that stored Ruth's special homemade chocolate chip cookies. As usual, I would ask for one and she would indulge me and the ritual would continue. She led the way as we walked through the tiny kitchen into the living room. Ruth would sit down on the well-worn couch, and I would find my spot on the floor sitting at her feet. While slowly eating my delicious morsel of goodness, I would listen to this aging woman share wisdom and life lessons I would never find in a book. I would absorb the stories of the unimaginable circumstances she found herself in, and each time she would share with me how God brought her through it.

Ruth captivated me with her intriguing stories that would one day become valuable lessons for me. Our history made her the perfect person to deliver the message to keep a journal. I had great respect for Ruth, and as I reflected on the power of this interaction, I knew deep down in my soul that she was telling me to "be prepared" because God was going to show up in my journey the same way he had shown up in hers. Every time I left Ruth's house, I couldn't believe one person could face so much pain, and I was even more captivated by how God helped her through it time and time again.

I continued to read a few pages of my journal on the long days I sat alone in my house. I quickly learned a few pages was all I could handle in one sitting. Each traumatic experience held memories that would, no doubt, take years or a lifetime to process. As I flipped through the pages and read a random excerpt, fear would grab its tight hold on me. The emotions were so raw. I was back there again as though no time had passed. As I continued to read, tears that represented the pain I was revisiting slowly dripped down my face and onto the pages of my journal. I was amazed at how often God rescued me and pulled me through when I couldn't imagine a way out of the devastating situation I found myself in. I broke out in goosebumps as I considered that what Ruth had said to me years earlier was clearly coming true. Deep down I knew that soon there would be a time for me to follow her second directive and share my story to encourage others the same way I had been encouraged when I sat at her feet and heard her stories.

Soon after I reflected on the amazing ways God had helped me, I found myself in a melancholy mood thinking about all the important dates and celebrations I had missed out on, but then, as quickly as those thoughts entered my mind, I had a feeling of contentment thinking about the chances I did get to celebrate. Even though there were fewer celebrations, they were more meaningful because I cherished each opportunity.

Some of the best moments I had, believe it or not, were with my doctor—that's right, my doctor. He dedicated his life to his work (me) and told me I could call him day or night. I couldn't put a price tag on his dedication to me, both inside the hospital and out. This type of relationship outside of just his amazing medical care was something I didn't take for granted. You see, my doctor and I had a common interest in sports. I was thankful for that mutual bond because he happened to sometimes receive tickets from the owners of a few Chicago professional sports teams.

On my birthday one year, I commemorated the special day with a routine that had become all too familiar. Instead of eating chocolate cake and opening presents, I recognized this day by throwing up my most recent meal, chewing on ice chips, and getting another round of chemo. Needless to say, I missed out on what should have been a joyous occasion. On that day, Dr. Nachman promised me that when I was feeling better he would take me to see my favorite baseball team, the Chicago Cubs (even though he was more of a White Sox fan). I treasure that memory to this day. Thankfully, with the help of my journal, I was able to capture the details so that my recollection of this special birthday stayed clear to me for years to come.

8/14/04

I didn't sleep well because I am very nauseous.... At 10:30 a.m., I met my doc on Randolph at his condo in the city overlooking Lake Michigan. On the drive down, I was holding back throwing up. Everything smelled because of the chemo. By the grace of God, I made it so we took the L to the game. I was supposed to stay out of the sun because of my medicine, so I wore my Cubs hat to stay shaded. I drank water throughout the game to keep hydrated. I learned everything was a million times worse if I'm not hydrated. We had the best seats. We sat in the fourth row directly behind home plate. I have never watched a game from there! It's like watching a different game. The ball shoots off the bat like a rocket and when it gets fouled back on the screen you think you're going to get nailed. Kerry Wood was pitching today. Man, does that ball move and man, does he throw smoke.

Later on we went swimming in his pool. It was in a huge glass dome. I had never seen anything like it. Afterward we went out on the balcony overlooking Lake Michigan. It was such a clear day that we could see Indiana and Michigan. We then took a walk to Buckingham Fountain. On the way there, across from his condo, was a cancer garden that was donated by a husband whose wife was a breast cancer survivor. I was really excited to see something like that. It really inspired me. When I am completely cured, I am going to go there with my family and plant my own flower in that cancer survivor garden.

As I slowly turned the pages, I came across another occasion when I had felt up to venturing out of my home. I had just finished a second round of chemo during my first bout with cancer when I decided to ask my nurse practitioner if it would be OK to travel to a friend's lake house with my dad to go fishing. She said yes, but there were some restrictions for my own safety. My blood count was too low to get in the water, but as long as I was careful I could ride in a boat. I figured fishing would be a great way to relax and celebrate having another round of treatment under my belt. She gave me the green light to go with my dad as long as I didn't bait the hook myself. My platelets were dangerously low, and if I cut myself with the hook there would be no way to stop the bleeding. My journal slowly released the sweet memories I thought were long gone.

7/26–7/28/04

Dad and I went to Lake Geneva! This was the first time I had gotten away all summer. It was great . . . oh, to relax. I would love to have a boat and a lake house someday.... It felt so good to stay in a house in the woods and be out on a boat, just enjoying the wonderful beauty of God's creation. It was like I didn't even have cancer. I was tired, but the great thing was that I forgot about it all.

My journal took me right back to that wonderful day with my dad. We must have found the right fishing hole because we pulled fish in left and right. Each time I reeled in a fish, he took the fish off the hook, threw it back, and baited the hook for me again. We caught mostly sunfish and bluegill, about thirty in all. I carried that enjoyable memory with me for days and weeks to come. My dad didn't often share tender words with me, but he did show me love through his actions. Baiting the hook and taking the fish off the hook throughout that afternoon was his way of saying "I love you, son," and I cherished it then and now. I continued reading. Once again, I was thankful my journal captured each emotion I felt in that exact moment.

It was great to spend time with Dad. I love him a lot and really appreciate him more now. Usually I'm just a jerk but he does so much for me, so many sacrifices—and now I'm starting to realize it. Thank God.

Reading about this amazing day with my dad strengthened my mental stamina, so I flipped to the next page and kept reading. I reflected on what happened next. I wanted to stay the weekend with my dad and continue fishing, but I couldn't because my dad needed to come home for a work meeting. Since the lake house was still available, my dad and I discussed returning to the lake for the weekend with the rest of my family after his meeting. I took advantage of being home and I decided to get my blood counts taken in hopes that they would have risen enough so I could go water skiing when we returned. I loved to be out on the water as often as I could. It was a peaceful environment for me. But I knew it was necessary for me to obtain my nurse practitioner's approval prior to making plans like these. My counts had risen to a safe enough level to get in the water. I was thrilled! I was thankful our friend gave us the keys to his house and boat that weekend so I could get away and seize the moment while I was up for this type of excursion.

The next day, I enjoyed being in Lake Geneva, Wisconsin, on a speedboat with Carrie and my immediate family. I strapped on my life jacket and jumped into the water. Once my water skis were on and the rope was in the correct position for takeoff, I signaled to my dad, who was driving, to give the boat some gas.

The momentum of being propelled on skis with the bright sun shining down on me, coupled with the warm wind and crisp water that blew directly in my face, was like experiencing a little slice of heaven. I stayed up on the skis for as long as possible and many minutes later I let go of the rope. As my body sank back into the cool water, so did my energy level. I was running on empty.

I needed help to get back into the boat due to sheer exhaustion. In fact, I was so tired that it was difficult to keep my eyes open, and my body shook terribly for the next few hours. My journal reminded me of this moment in time when falling asleep after a long day of fun in the sun was a reality for me.

I slept until about nine o'clock when my dad woke me up to go home. A trip on skis sent me into a deep slumber. Cancer wears you out. You know how when you are overtired, you dream a lot? Well, I dream practically every time I sleep—no matter where or when. If I'm sleeping, I'm dreaming!

The memory of that day opened the floodgates to the emotions I experienced at the time. The somewhat brief celebration of life did so much for me. Finishing another three days of treatment brought me one step closer to the finish line, and that was reason to celebrate! I relived that moment in the sun time and time again and today, even as I reflect now, the experience still brings me joy.

After reading and reflecting on these small jewels of joy that were sprinkled in throughout my cancer journey, I realized these memories were priceless. Thinking back, I recall yearning for more celebratory occasions to help me get through my dark days and around that time, I remember thanking God and asking him, if it was his will, to please give me more chances to celebrate life. Shortly after I had that thought, Joel called me. Our college soccer coach had invited us to come watch a private scrimmage for the United States Men's Soccer Team as they prepared for the World Cup. Coincidence? I think not. The field they were playing at was where I played my last collegiate soccer game. Tears began to stream down my face as I listened to his voice. I was flooded with raw emotions. The memories rewound the clock to a time when I was a sought-after college athlete. Now I was going to struggle just to get out of the car to see the best soccer players in the United States play on the field where I played my last game.

The drive to the field made me quickly realize how far I still had to go on the road to recovery. It was hard for my eyes to keep up with the changing scenery at 40 miles per hour. The movement made me sick to my stomach. By the time we arrived at the field, I struggled out of the car and had to find a place in the shade to watch the scrimmage. As I watched, memories went through my mind of the last soccer game I played and I reflected on how grateful I was to be there that day. After the game, I went up to Brian McBride, a player on the team I had met years ago, to see if he remembered me. Receiving encouragement from the captain of the team went a long way. I struggled back to the car, made my way back home and, upon arrival, collapsed on my bed. The trip wore me out for the next few days, but I focused on the fact that it was totally worth it.

Making progress in adjusting my attitude was painful, but the hard work I put into correcting my course always paid off and brought me toward feeling hopeful again. I knew that this persistent, positive attitude was crucial to my survival.

"God is our refuge and strength, an ever-present help in times of trou-

ble" (Psalm 46:1). In times of desperation, it can become incomprehensible to embrace this claim, but much like the calmness found in the center of a hurricane, it is possible for us to find protection in the middle of it. That is where we find peace. Once we have this revelation, it can become easier to start and end each day with a hopeful attitude which emboldens us and makes it quite possible to conquer fear while knowing we're living directly in the eye of the storm.

Reflection Questions

1. Who can you encourage by sharing and asking them about things they are thankful for?

2. How have you seen thankfulness keep you encouraged during a difficult time?

CHAPTER 15

LOVE IS POWER

&

Love is an amazingly multifaceted word, seen clearly by the many words for love in the Greek language. *Eros* is used to define the type of love a person has when they are physically attracted to someone. The word *erotic* stems from this type of love. Another word the Greeks use to define love is *philia*, which signifies the kind of love found in a close friendship. The city of brotherly love, Philadelphia, derives its name from the meaning of this word. Both of these types of love are meant to bring forth an emotional reaction in a person. Yet another type of love is meant to move beyond an emotion—*agape*. This is the deepest form of love which moves people to act on behalf of others. This expression of love can be seen through the eyes of someone who exhibits caring and concern for others, and will deeply develop from knowing Christ.

Agape moves us beyond ourselves; it can set us free from darkness and remove the power cancer has over us. In the absence of this love, all light fades from our lives and darkness closes in around us. But when unconditional love is given to us in our most devastating moments, it has the power to alter any situation we face. Each act of love can brighten our space like a perpetual, glimmering light that chases away the darkness.

***

September finally ended and October arrived with much antici-
pated joy. After two months of being chained to an intolerable IV,
my nurse came to my home to disconnect me from this unwelcome
intruder. After she set me free, we exchanged wide-eyed smiles and
went our separate ways. No more daily visits, just weekly check-ins
and appointments when needed. Each step I took down the creaking
stairs from my bedroom to the first floor left me feeling more stable
and confident. With a skip in my step, I decided to venture outside for
a walk around the block. I inhaled deeply and my lungs filled with re-
freshing cool air. I suddenly found it easier to breathe than it had been
for months before. The earthy smell of autumn was in the air. The rus-
set and goldenrod leaves were gently falling to their final resting spot. I
was mesmerized by this common experience that most people took for
granted and thought to myself, *Oh, how colorful this journey can be!*

In my story I found beauty, especially in what people did for me.
Shortly after I was diagnosed, a group of people put a care package
together for me. This act of kindness caused me to break down and cry.
The care package, full of items I needed and enjoyed, symbolized that
I wasn't going to fight through this journey alone. Even more so, that
small expression of care was also the starting point for me to realize
how important it would be for me to accept the help of others.

Previously, I had taken pride in succeeding in tasks on my own.
Now I needed a strong team to cheer me on every step of the way, in
the same way a rookie marathoner needs encouragement to finish their
maiden race.

When I was well enough to begin the recuperation process from
home, I laid upstairs on the couch passing time with mindless televi-
sion viewing. No matter how exhausted I was, each afternoon I repeatedly checked my watch to see if it was 1:00 p.m. yet—that's when the

mail arrived. When the clock struck one, I would muster up as much energy as possible to sit on the edge of the couch. Once the dizziness subsided, I would stand up slowly and make my way to the staircase. I hobbled toward the wooden banister and looked down the stairs, taking a moment to catch my breath in anticipation of my next step. I would slowly descend the staircase, sliding my hand down the banister to provide stability to my precarious balance. At the bottom of the stairs, I would pause again to catch my breath. Grabbing the nearest wall to maintain my balance, I would then walk through the dining room toward the front door. I vividly remember the feeling of anticipation as I turned the door knob, wondering, *Would this be the day someone remembered me?* In years past, I wouldn't have thought twice about this rudimentary task, but today and every day since that first care package arrived, I looked forward to retrieving whatever might come in the mail that would symbolize the idea that someone cared for me that day. My routine was always the same. I would reach into the mailbox and pull out a stack of envelopes and quickly sift through all the mail. Each week for two years, I pulled out a card with my name on it from someone named Judy whom I'd never met. With that special note in hand and my energy depleted, I would place the rest of the mail back inside the box for my family to retrieve later and begin to make the long trek back up the stairs to the place that beckoned my return.

It would usually take me longer to get back to the couch from the mailbox, having to stop more frequently to catch my breath. But amazingly enough, the second leg of the journey didn't seem as painful with the anticipation of reading a letter of encouragement. This was yet another reminder of how much farther a person can go with a supportive team of people cheering them on.

Although the round-trip journey from the couch to the mailbox wore me out for the rest of the day, it was worth it to see what was inside that card. The simple task of opening the envelope was another challenge because of my trembling hands, a side effect of the ever-present lethal drugs running through my veins. But once I saw the content within the envelope, I never regretted the effort I took to get it. Each card held a special message that inspired me to persevere. A funny joke would bring a smile to my face, and a Bible verse would uplift my spirits for days. Sometimes written in the card were four short, simple words: "I'm praying for you." It was as if God hand delivered the letters—the message was always exactly *what* I needed exactly *when* I needed it. If I was weak, it was a message about strength; if I was heartbroken, it was a message about peace. If I was lacking faith, it contained another one of God's promises. Each card let me know I was truly not alone.

These cards of encouragement brought to mind a special person whose spiritual life made a difference for me on my journey. From a young age, I looked up to my grandfather as a role model in my life. He was extremely loving, always led by example, and offered wise advice. I remember one day in particular when I woke up from a nap in my hospital bed. As I opened my eyes, to my surprise, I saw him sitting quietly in a chair in the corner of my room. He said hello and proceeded to page through a book he was reading. Reading books was not an uncommon practice for him as a lifelong learner, teacher, and pastor. Eventually it dawned on me that he was highlighting verses in the Bible my Aunt Kathy had given me for confirmation in seventh grade. Growing up, that book had sat on a bookshelf collecting dust most of the time. That day, my grandpa highlighted all the verses in my Bible that referenced the words hope, faith, strength, and peace, and then he encouraged me by reading aloud each verse he had highlighted. He read about hope in Lamentations 3:25–27—*"The Lord is good to those whose hope is in him, to the one who seeks him; it is good to wait quietly for the salvation of the Lord. It is good for a man to bear the yoke while he is young.*" And then faith, as my grandpa knew it, was explained to me when he read from Hebrews 11:1—*"Now faith is being sure of what you hope for and certain of what you do not see."* Next, he shared his definition of strength by reading from Philippians 4:13—*"I can do all things through Christ who gives me strength."* Finally, my grandpa read to me from Proverbs 14:30 to teach me about the true meaning of peace—*"A heart at peace gives life to the body, but envy rots the bones."* After reading the verses aloud to me, my grandfather walked over to my bedside and gave me a hug, looked into my eyes, and said, "Philip, Grandma and I love you and so does your Heavenly Father." He then placed the Bible on the tray located on the side of my bed and walked out. There was power in his presence, and I was thankful he made the trip to Chicago from St. Louis to encourage me. Over the next few weeks, I paged through my Bible to see the verses he highlighted and committed them to memory. When I was too sick to open my eyes, those verses ran through my head and sunk into the depths of my heart. God's promises to me brought victory over cancer and became my source of strength and peace.

When I faced death, I knew I should pray diligently and continuously. When my energy was depleted and I was weighed down with grief, God used Carrie to encourage me. In my worried state of mind, she would use the Bible as her bedrock to show me God's truth. Her Bible was worn and tattered because of all the time she spent growing her intimate relationship with God. Cancer always had a way of pulling me into the pit of despair, while Carrie was the extraordinary example of how to stay positive when faced with uncertainties. If she cried, she rarely did it around me as she knew I needed her to be a stable force throughout the journey. Every person needs a warrior like Carrie.

She taught me how to pray during my weakest moments and reminded me of God's promise to us in James 4:8, *"Draw near to God, and he will draw near to you."*

Taking God at his word, in desperation, I called on him and he answered. It was awkward for me at first, much like initial conversations on a blind date. But I continued on, "God, I know you are listening, so I'm just going to talk to you." There was nothing polished or eloquent about my praying, only words straight from my heart. I told God how I felt—whether angry, joyful, or sad—and asked him for help.

It takes time to cultivate a relationship with anybody, and this relationship was no different. But as the months passed, I couldn't imagine what life was like before discovering the type of intimacy I had with God. He was as close to me as a best friend could be. I focused on just being still and knowing that he was a loving God. How amazing it was to learn over and over again that he always listens and is always there for me.

***

Most of us have heard that there is more joy in giving than in receiving. For those of us who have experienced this joy, we know it to be true. We give to others with the intention of brightening their day, but soon realize through the act of giving that we are twice as blessed in return. Love, when given unconditionally, is the greatest superpower, the ultimate encourager, and, when activated, can breathe life into a person and pull them out of the depths of despair. This is love: the most powerful four-letter word in the dictionary.

Reflection Questions

1. Is there a time in your life when you have received unconditional love, and it altered your situation?
2. What verses have meant a lot for you in your journey throughout

life? What verses have you committed to memory?

CHAPTER 16

FORGET THE MESS

∽

Although we may differ from one another as to how much mess we can handle, we all suffer from the same life-threatening condition called sin. If left unaddressed, it will severely limit us in life and potentially destroy us for eternity. Thankfully, we can clean up the mess we've made so death doesn't get the final say.

***

As I would lay in my hospital bed, my mind would wander as I thought about the true meaning of life. All the signs around me on the journey confirmed for me that life was no accident. I also discovered that one body system couldn't function on its own—they all needed to work in tandem for me to survive. In the stillness of my existence, I saw too many miracles that became unexplained events to write off as coincidences.

As I contemplated the possibility of my impending death, I knew more decisively than ever that there wasn't anything I could do to save myself. No amount of stored up good works that I did in my past could rescue me and guarantee my eternity. Like a beating drum, the precious words of Jesus would echo through my mind, reassuring me that *"unless one is born again, he cannot see the kingdom of God"* (John 3:3).

God's Word presented example after example of messed up people like me whom he saved and then used for his purposes. In the confines of my hospital bed, I worshiped him, and as I did, my desire to be used in a powerful way to impact his kingdom on Earth grew.

When I was lying awake feeling nauseous, struggling to get comfortable from the pain, ominous voices would enter my head, forcing me to recoil at each and every thought: "You are going to die. This is going to kill you. You are not going to make it." These words served as a reminder that I was in a war, battling for my life. Thankfully God's Word taught me that I had power over these atrocious demons who were trying to take up residence within me. All that really mattered was the knowledge that my loving and ever-present God was undoubtedly in control. Even though I was too weak and feeble to move at times on this journey, I learned one truth that was undeniable: I could always stand firm on God's rock-solid promises. When the unrelenting attacks came in the middle of the night and I felt miserably alone and defeated, I would reach out to my God and, suddenly, the strength of David fighting off Goliath would come to me. Deep within my soul, I would shout back to those demons: "In the name of Jesus, get behind me Satan! Get out of my head! Get out of my room! Get out of this house! Go back to where you belong!" After engaging in this intense battle, exhaustion would ultimately settle in, and I fell asleep peacefully.

As I mentioned earlier, I had an enormous epiphany when I realized that cancer was no longer a battle to fight on my own. I had the Creator of the world fighting with me and for me. God used well-informed and knowledgeable doctors to help make decisions about my care, nurses who worked alongside these doctors and showed their compassion for me on a daily basis, caregivers who never left my side, and life-saving medications to shepherd me throughout my journey. I had another "aha" moment when it occurred to me that almost everything I desired in life before my diagnosis had been lost somewhere along the journey, and at the time it had truly grieved me. However, I realized that as my health had declined, much of what I was desperately trying to hold onto needed to be released as well. It took a major jolt like cancer to sever those wants and desires, but more importantly, throughout this experience, I began to understand how grand life could be without them. Before cancer, I thought my purpose in life was to exist day to day, making the most out of each selfish moment. But, ironically, throughout this long and arduous journey, with death knocking at my door, I ended up finding my true purpose in life.

Now I knew deep down in my heart that the greatest purpose of my life was no longer to beat cancer—it was to surrender to God's will and be content each day, no matter the outcome. Oh, how liberating this declaration was for me! Then, just like soldiers marching to the rhythm of their battle cry, God's Word came to me as a triumphant proclamation: *"Do not be anxious about anything, but in everything by prayer and supplication with thanksgiving let your requests be made known to God. And the peace of God, which surpasses all understanding, will guard your hearts and your minds in Christ Jesus"* (Philippians 4:6–7). Having this unimaginable peace was a monumental contributor to my positive state of mind. In fact, it was around this time that I had an insightful revelation and began to clearly see that having cancer really wasn't going to be my ultimate story. On the contrary, God used my sickness as a way of making known to me that there was so much more to tell than the unraveling story of my cancer journey.

During my stem-cell transplant, I was at my weakest moment and it was then that I hit my breaking point. I remember crying out to God and pleading with him in total desperation, "If it's time for me to go to Heaven, I'm ready. But if it isn't my time, I promise to devote the rest of my life to you and what you have planned for me." This was my "all-in" moment. It took death knocking at my door to finally give up any hope that I could beat this cruel disease by myself. In return, I made the best choice of my life and decided to put all my hope in Jesus. *"For God so loved the world that he gave his one and only son that whoever believes in him will not perish but have eternal life"* (John 3:16). Knowing this in my head and heart unequivocally made salvation my starting point, not only my end. Jesus was now Lord of my life. Believing this truth sealed my eternity and, at the same time, limited my worries.

***

Cancer and chemotherapy can leave a person's body a mess. In sickness and during our darkest moments we often cry out for someone to rescue us from our suffering and pain. But, for those of us who understand that our body on this Earth is only temporary, a sense of undeniable peace takes place knowing that Jesus can save us from the greatest cancer this world has ever known—sin. In Luke 23:42, the criminal being crucified next to Jesus said, *"Jesus, remember me when you come into your kingdom."* Jesus reassured the man by responding, *"Today you will be with me in paradise."* Salvation through Jesus is for everyone and all that is needed is an open heart and an invitation for him to come in. Our lives on Earth are temporary, but eternity is forever. There are no magic words. All it takes is simply telling Jesus you're sorry for your sins, thanking him for dying for you, and asking his forgiveness. When we call on Jesus, the mess we created through our sin is wiped away, leaving us perfectly clean in God's eyes. Our name is then added to the book of life as a survivor of the greatest cancer of all.

Reflection Questions

1. What is your story of how God saved you? Who or what did he use to draw you to himself?

2. Have you considered that your greatest purpose in life is to surrender to God's will and be content each day, no matter the out come? How does that resonate with you?

CHAPTER 17

COMFORTED TO COMFORT OTHERS

Once we experience hopelessness on our cancer journey, we understand at the deepest level that others may have experienced it too. When our bodies are broken and our spirits are crushed, the battle can be unbearable. When we see others in situations like ours, we're sure that, just like us, none of them ever wanted to be there. Who is going to come alongside others with cancer to give them hope and help them walk the difficult road they don't want to travel? Pondering such a question can move us from seeing ourselves as a simple bystander to someone who has a purpose in this world. Once this internal exchange takes place, it's only a matter of time before something needs to be done.

During my recovery process, I set bite-size goals. First I wanted to sit up on the edge of my bed. Then I set a goal to make it to the bathroom by myself. Eventually, with the help of a nurse or family member, I made it into the hallway. Then with my IV pole in tow I set a goal to make it around the hospital floor. Each day I grew stronger and made it a little further. I paused at each open door to catch my breath. I saw two-year-olds confined to their beds with enough tubing connected to them to stretch down the hallway. I saw five- and ten-year-olds sitting in bed awake and alone. And the sight of teenagers and countless adults with nobody by their side to comfort or strengthen them brought tears to my eyes. It didn't matter if they were two or ninety-two, the look on each of their faces told their story of anguish. Eerily, the disheartening images I saw on those walks haunt me to this day and have become a constant reminder of what life is like for people dealing with cancer.

Those images of suffering were seared into my heart and mind. I felt broken from my own circumstances, but seeing others in similar situations all alone devastated me even more than the cancer itself. I've heard that if you truly want to know how someone feels, you should walk a mile in their shoes. Well, I had a chance to walk in the shoes of so many people before me who found themselves in this place of despair. I knew right then and there that my cancer would not be wasted. Suddenly, it hit me—*"He comforts us in all our troubles so that we can comfort others. When they are troubled, we will be able to give them the same comfort God has given us"* (2 Corinthians 1:4). It became clear to me that people of all ages who are fighting for their life want to keep their dignity and need someone to comfort them and help them carry their awful load.

A fire was set in my soul. Something had to be done. At that point, I was in no shape to do anything except make eye contact and send a friendly smile. In that moment, I knew in the depths of my being that if I was blessed with restored health and if I was given the opportunity to help fellow cancer warriors in the future, I would do so—no matter what it would cost me.

Throughout my journey I experienced unmet needs and I felt called to help people who experienced the same. I didn't know how or what I would do, but I knew I was called to be a part of the solution. One day, a friend called my dad after hearing that I wanted to help people. Inspired by an organization called Joni and Friends that helps the disabled, he suggested that I'd need a name if I wanted to help people.

He suggested I call it "Phil's Friends." With that nugget of an idea and the support of family by my side, the beginning of an organization was born.

One day, while my father was visiting me in the hospital, a few of his business friends showed up at my bedside. One friend was an attorney, and he brought information on how to start a 501(c)(3) not-for-profit organization. Together, they walked me through the process, but I didn't have the energy to do much more than listen. In fact, I was so physically weak and shaky that when the time came, I needed help picking up my hand to sign the necessary paperwork. But, in that moment, Phil's Friends was officially put into motion!

At the close of 2005, I finally finished up radiation and was declared cancer free for the second time. I threw a big "cancer free" party to celebrate. Life is too short not to party! At the conclusion of the party, I passed out a letter I had written to express my love to each person in attendance, share how my life had changed for the better, and conclude with a vision to "get in the game" and support others facing cancer. Being diagnosed with cancer put life into perspective and lit a fire beneath me to get out there and do something. This included being more of an open book in life and sharing my feelings. Today, it's not uncommon for me to tear up and voice to a loved one, "If today is my last day, I want you to know how grateful I am for you and how much I love you."

Preparing to re-enter back into society was challenging. It was a year-long process to build up stamina after my transplant as I suffered from severe short-term memory loss and overall weakness. I was used to focusing solely on my health, but once my health no longer required my full-time attention, I had freedom and, although limited, more energy for other activities. That included learning about what it takes to create a startup organization. As my physical health recovered and I reflected on how far I'd already come, my appreciation for the spiritual and emotional growth that took place during such a silent period of my life grew even more. New dreams were within reach, and dreams I had let go of while I focused on surviving began to resurface. Going back to work, marrying Carrie, and having children of my own were once again realistic dreams for me.

In March 2006, while continuing to formulate in my mind what it would take to make Phil's Friends a viable organization, I returned to the classroom once again to teach fourth grade. My students were thankful to see me, and I was equally grateful to see them. Although I was thrilled to be back, it left me exhausted. I quickly discovered that the key to moving forward was to live in the present, accept help when it was offered, and take time to look back to where I'd been to continually remind myself how far I'd already come.

Spending time with my class further fueled the energy to support others with cancer. Sometimes my students would brainstorm with me about ways to help people who were in need. They were passionate about helping their teacher and soon that passion was harnessed to help others too. Word spread from the students to their families and each act of love given out to someone on the cancer journey set us up to be an explosive force. The students helped make cards and came up with ideas to help as many people as possible. My family and I assembled the first care package—a handmade card along with some small toys, games, and a children's Bible—and delivered it to a special five-year-old girl, my friend Jenna.

A month later, Melissa, the mom of one of the students in my class, approached me after school and asked me my favorite color. I thought that was an odd question, but I told her baby blue. The following week, she and other parents surprised me with baby blue wristbands that said "Phil's Friends." The students sold the wristbands and raised $133. This launched the very first Phil's Friends fundraiser. With the money collected, we set up a bank account and Carrie and I had a crucial conversation that led us to deciding how to be faithful with every penny. My immediate family and close friends rallied around the cause to make our dream a reality. Weston, my good friend and the college roommate, stepped forward and offered to plan and execute a walkathon to raise awareness and necessary funding. The planning committee met consistently in my classroom in the evenings. My family and I took trips to Walmart to buy care package items. Soon our vehicles couldn't fit what we needed, so we borrowed eight-passenger vans. We took trips to the dollar store to purchase as many items as we could and filled the van until the doors could barely shut. That first year, the organization continued to grow and we were able to help over one hundred deserving families. The more we loved others, the more God continued to expand our reach.

Reflection Questions

1. What dreams do you have that you've either had to put on hold or could pursue with limited energy?

2. How can you creatively support people who have been through things similar to you?

CHAPTER 18

HIS PLAN IS BEST

✥

On June 17, 2006, I woke up in a hotel room in Mattoon, Illinois. It was my wedding day. Thoughts swirled through my mind as I tried to wrap my head around the reality of it all. After everything we had been through together, I couldn't believe this day was finally here. As I stood looking out the window at the corn fields, I shook my head in disbelief thinking about how the past few years unfolded. Why is it that we often fight so hard against situations in our lives and only later come to realize that what we fought against was actually best for us? Here I was in a town I hadn't wanted to spend time in, getting married to a girl I'd never wanted to meet. I finally understood the plan I fought so hard against was always best for me.

I took some deep breaths and began the process of preparing for this remarkable moment in my life. Thankfully, I was used to centering myself each morning, one of the many gifts I still carry with me from my cancer journey. My daily routine of showering, shaving, and preparing for the day took on new meaning as I finished the process by putting on a formal tux. I took one final look in the mirror and saw a man quite different from the person who first met Carrie four years ago—a better man.

Later that day, as I stood at the altar waiting for the ceremony to begin, anticipation of what was to come raced through my mind. I heard the gentle, metallic, sweet sound of a harp drifting throughout the church rafters before I actually saw the person who was plucking the strings with precision. When I turned and spotted our friend Jen playing the instrument, I reminisced about the time I tried to break out of the hospital to attend her and Ryan's wedding only to be reprimanded by the nurses as they saw me heading for the exits with blood dripping down my body. I grew increasingly emotional looking at my mom, dad, and other loved ones who sacrificed so much for me. When I looked at my younger siblings, I remembered the fears they had of losing their older brother. My emotions continued to rise as I saw all who were in attendance. For Carrie and me, it was a true representation of the community that had rallied around us over the past few years. I took a glance at the officiant—my grandfather, the godly man who filled me with Scripture verses during my darkest moments, knew all that it took for me to be standing there that day.

The pinnacle of my emotions came when the church doors opened and I saw Carrie standing there in her white dress, locking arms with her dad. To me, she was undeniably the most beautiful bride in the world. I savored each and every moment as they slowly walked up the aisle, and I knew right there and then that the woman I was about to marry was everything to me. I held it together as she and her father made their way to the front of the church. Once they reached the altar, I gently held Carrie's hands and told her how beautiful she looked and whispered the words I planned to say to her for the rest of our lives: "I love you." We then slowly turned to face my grandfather.

During my grandfather's heartfelt message, he let Carrie know what a blessing she was to me, and if not for her dedication, this special occasion would not be happening. With tears streaming down my face, I shook my head in agreement and held her hand tighter to affirm my feelings. He then continued, "Carrie and Phil, it's pure joy for me to see the way you look into each other's eyes, and I'm enjoying the view so much that I think it's only appropriate for you both to turn around and face everyone so that they too can see the happiness that radiates from your faces." In our marriage, we knew what we were signing up for, especially when we took our vows to stay together in sickness and in health. Those words had such profound meaning to us, as I'm also sure it did for every person in the church that day.

As we started our life together, our dream of expanding our family came true as well. Preparing the nursery took on special meaning for Carrie and me, as it does for many first-time parents. I'll never forget the time when my nurse Kelly called to check in on us to see how preparations were going. What she said left me speechless. This woman God used to take care of me while I was in the hospital, and who helped give me the opportunity to be a father, offered us a crib, which was the final piece we needed to finish the room. Every time I saw the crib, I choked up. It symbolized to me how much care I needed during the time I spent in the hospital just a short time ago. Ironically, this gift would be used to provide for a new life who would need a lot of care from me.

In April 2013, Graham was born. I remember holding Graham for the first time. I wept and grew increasingly thankful as I was brought back to the moment Doctor Nachman told me to go to the sperm bank before my treatment started. At the time, I couldn't truly appreciate the significance of his suggestion, but it was through in vitro fertilization that this miracle occurred. Hudson followed a few years later.

As the clock plays forward in our lives, we never know what God has in store for us. All I know is that the more life goes on, the more we can come to expect the unexpected as we put our trust in Jesus. Having our own children changed our lives, but I never expected to one day tell my friends and family that my wife was pregnant with another man's baby. Let me explain: Carrie saw a well-deserving family with a need and felt called to be a surrogate for this couple. My diagnosis with cancer made her a perfect candidate because of her history with in vitro fertilization. In the midst of my wife's desire to pour out her love to others, she discovered that she was called to be a blessing to another family who desperately wanted a little one to love.

***

You've heard the saying, "Where there's a will, there's a way." While this sentiment can be comforting to think about during a person's cancer journey, it doesn't always tell the full story. We may possess the will, but we cannot always make a way. Among God's people, a greater truth is voiced when we say, "If it is God's will, he will make a way." Don't forget that Jesus declared, *"I am the way, the truth, and the life"* (John 14:6). Two thousand years ago the Way comforted Paul and the disciples so they could comfort others. The same Messiah is in the business of comforting us in our sufferings so that we, too, can comfort others. Today we can move forward boldly because God knows what is best for us and he alone knows the rest of our story.

Reflection Questions

1. What things have you fought against in life that ended up being what was actually best for you?

2. How can you see God's hand in your story through the people he's put in your life?

CHAPTER 19

CREATING A MOVEMENT

⊱

Each of us can be inspired by a new idea, but pulling the trigger to get started can be the hardest part. If we're not careful, we can talk ourselves out of anything, especially when others around us don't sense the calling we have to move forward. These naysayers come to us with an assortment of reasons as to why it can't be done. I believe if change came easily, more people would be excited about it. At the end of the day, life isn't meant to be easy.

If we cannot envision a better tomorrow, we can end up being locked in a cage with our own circumstances. So, when we catch a vision and hear God's calling for our life, it's paramount that we act on it. We either move with the torch in our hand for others to see or the fire will burn out. Baby steps, together with a truckload of courage, will set us on the right path. And our passion coupled with bold vision can be a contagious fuel.

***

After a lot of sweat and tears, Phil's Friends officially became recognized by the government as a 501(c)(3) organization in November 2006. By then, the Phil's Friends mission to bring hope and support to those affected by cancer was well underway. In a few short years, the organization turned into a movement. We continued to support people in the same way I was supported when I was sick—providing a loving community to help meet cancer patients' physical, spiritual, and emotional needs.

When Phil's Friends was in its embryonic stage, I continued my teaching career while juggling the operations of running a new business. I recruited three parents of students in my fourth-grade class and provided them with keys to my house so they could venture into my basement and assemble care packages for individuals with cancer. They recruited other committed and passionate volunteers. During this time, I focused my efforts on helping friends with cancer. Recruiting and empowering passionate helpers to move the mission forward also became a priority for me.

My mentor, Charlie, encouraged me to take advantage of all opportunities that would help move the mission forward. And one soon presented itself: we were given a chance to have our first booth at a concert to raise awareness. My family and I showed up with a few care packages and handouts to pass out. We had no idea at the time that this event would put a snowball effect in motion that would open up doors for Phil's Friends in a variety of places.

After setting up our booth, Ed, the concert promoter, welcomed us. He shared how grateful he was for our mission and how encouraged he was by my story. He was so inspired that he asked me if I would be willing to speak to the crowd before the concert started. Saying I was very reluctant to agree is an understatement. The thought of speaking in front of a large crowd made me break out in hives! Nevertheless, I followed Charlie's advice and agreed.

Just before it was time to get ready to go on stage, I found myself in the bathroom not feeling well. I was a nervous wreck. I hid in that bathroom and didn't come out until I was sure I'd missed the opportunity to speak. When I thought the coast was clear, I opened the door and, to my surprise,

Ed was walking briskly down the hallway with a few radio station emcees. He called out, "Phil, just in time! Follow us." This pushed my panic button! We quickly walked behind the stage and Ed said, "Phil, you have two minutes. I want you to go last, tell your story, and introduce the music artist." My heart was racing when I walked onto the stage and greeted the 3,000 people staring back at me. I tried not to trip over my own two feet as I grabbed the microphone as though it was my new best friend.

As I'd learned in my cancer journey, the best thing for me to do in moments like those was to pray and ask that my Lord give me the words. By the way the crowd reacted, I was sure every word I spoke was an undeniable gift from God. When I was finished, the crowd cheered and I walked off the stage feeling very relieved—and surprised that it went so well.

The more I continued to help others, the more confident I became. I developed a can-do attitude, knowing all that was required was to say yes and go. How freeing it became to have the assurance that God met me wherever I was meant to be and guided me the rest of the way! Soon I was invited to open more concerts, and every time I went on stage, God gave me the perfect message to give my audience. Around this time, a local radio station contacted me and allowed me to spread my message through the airwaves.

Over the next few years, the demand for our services increased as awareness grew. Soon the supplies spilled over from my basement into my garage and then began to take over the first floor of my house. Eventually, I hit a breaking point. Although it's nice that the volunteers can let your dog out while you're teaching, there comes a time when you can't give everyone a key to your house.

Living in this crossroads for awhile led Carrie and me to a pivotal conversation. I'll never forget that moment when Carrie asked, "Phil, do you feel called to teach twenty-eight children in a classroom setting the rest of your life, or to set up an organization that could potentially support millions of people one day?" I knew both were worthy and important callings, but I also knew deep down inside that teaching in one classroom wasn't the type of work God was calling me to do. This realization ignited an undeniable passion in my heart and the answer became clear: I decided I would leave my teaching position in order to focus all my energy on Phil's Friends.

Many people close to me verbalized that I was insane for leaving my job with no guarantee of an income. Plus, to make matters worse, our nation was right in the middle of a financial recession, the likes of which had not been seen in decades. If I had listened solely to these individuals who challenged my decision, I could have been paralyzed. When I added everything up from a human perspective, it didn't make sense to leave my job with nothing waiting for me. I was starting to lose my confidence, but thankfully I had two wise mentors in their seventies who showed me the way and taught me what it would take to become an effective leader. Rich and Charlie were full of wisdom, and during one of our early morning meetings, Charlie looked me in the eyes and said, "Phil, I think it's time for you to step out and follow your calling. The signs are all around you." Rich agreed with his sentiments. These special men impacted my thinking on life and helped me to see that we were not created to look at God from our worldly perspective; rather, we were created to see the world from a godly point of view. Soon enough I would have proof of my own that God multiplies our faithfulness. I just had to be patient to see how he would work out all the details!

When I finally left my teaching job in 2009, it wasn't easy. At the time I first started thinking about leaving my teaching job, Carrie and I were new parents with a hefty mortgage and two car payments. To make matters more challenging, Phil's Friends had no money in the bank to support an employee because we'd made the decision to put all the funding back into the organization to help those in need. But I left my job anyway. I wasn't afraid or apprehensive about my decision because I knew from past experience that the ground beneath my feet was more durable to walk on when following God's plan for me.

I didn't have to wait long to see how my life would soon change with my new outlook. A generous individual stepped forward and offered us free space in the community for ninety days after a ten-minute phone conversation. We later met in person so he could better understand the mission, and afterward, the space was offered to us as long as we needed it—free of charge! This is not to say that the journey was always easy. Very rarely did it go as I had planned, but in spite of some of the setbacks, I received daily encouragement reminding me that *"we can make our plans, but the Lord determines our steps"* (Proverbs 16:9).

At the next Phil's Friends Board meeting, I shared my decision to leave the teaching profession and the reasons behind it. It was clear that the organization was starting to burst at the seams and it could no longer function without full-time leadership. Also, through my personal observations, I knew it was not feasible for my health or marriage to hold up trying to balance teaching and the demands of growing this mission. But the Board looked at the resources in the bank and made the hard decision not to hire me until the bank balance was built up and the organization was more mature. Needless to say, after that meeting, I found myself in a place of deep despondency. I desperately wanted to follow God's will, but I was unsure of what he wanted me to do. When I stepped in the house that night and informed Carrie of the disappointing news, she said, "Phil, maybe it's a good thing. Now you have to get out there and tell your story." She was right and that's just what I did.

Within a month, seventy volunteers helped move inventory into our new space. Stepping foot into my new office put me in a euphoric mood, and I couldn't wait to get started! As we began to unpack the boxes, the office phone rang. Hearing that sound for the first time truly left me feeling downright giddy with excitement. The first call came from the Chicago Bears asking me if I would share my story before a Monday Night Football game against the Philadelphia Eagles. To my surprise, over sixty players and coaches showed up to hear me speak. I continued to share my story with as many people as possible, at times accepting three or four speaking engagements a day. Eventually, through much hard work and determination, there were enough resources for the Board of Directors to hire me as a full-time employee.

As word continued to spread, new volunteers would show up on a daily basis to put together care packages and make cards. I welcomed each volunteer who walked through the front door with a friendly smile and an extended hand to show my appreciation. One day I greeted a new volunteer, Judy. With passion in her voice, she mentioned that a friend told her Phil's Friends sends cards to the sick, so she decided to come in and see how she could help. The emotion in Judy's voice reached new heights when she explained that she'd been sending week-ly cards to the sick for decades.

When she told me her last name, chills went through my body. Standing in front of me was the woman who had sent me a card each week throughout my journey, and she had no idea that the reason we support thousands of people today with cards is because she first loved me! Tears began to stream down my face as I shared this revelation with her. She was surprised to learn how much her support had been a lifeline to me and had given me hope for the long, grueling journey of cancer. A few years later, Judy was diagnosed with breast cancer herself, and we supported her in the same way she had supported me.

Eventually, our little 800-square-foot office couldn't keep up with the demand. In 2012 we expanded and established the first Phil's Friends Hope Center where volunteers of all ages served in groups making cards and putting packages together. Since its inception, and with the help of thousands of volunteers, Phil's Friends has created tens of thousands of care packages and sent more than a million cards for cancer patients around the world. Each package and card is a reminder to people that hope is stronger than cancer.

A year later, I met Carolyn. She felt compelled to get involved after hearing me on the radio. As a leukemia survivor, her heart's desire was to reach out and love the patients on the hospital floor where she was treated. We became fast friends and together we established the Hope to Hospitals program with a vision of engaging an army of volunteers to meet people where they are in their cancer journey. This program is stationed at local hospitals where we provide care packages, encouragement, and prayer. Sadly, Carolyn's leukemia returned a few years after the program was established and she passed away. I miss her dearly and so many other friends we've lost on this journey. But Carolyn is proof that every story matters and that it only takes one willing individual with a story to change the world. As a result of her efforts, even in her absence from us, thousands of people with cancer will now receive support every year. And it goes even further! Carolyn had a dream of planting the first volunteer Hope Center in the state of Indiana. Even though she didn't get to see it come to pass, her vision came true. Within a year of her death, thanks to her best friend Judy along with her family and friends, a volunteer Hope Center in Crown Point, Indiana was established in Carolyn's honor.

Moses was a man full of doubt until God proclaimed with absolute assurance, *"I will be with you,"* every step of the way (Exodus 3:12). Moses learned not to be afraid to step out in faith when knowing he was doing God's work and will for his people. His life lesson could also resonate with each of us: it doesn't depend on what we do, but how God chooses to equip us to do it. And if we stumble along the way— no worries. These mishaps can become part of our life lessons when we keep in mind that we learn as much from our failures as we do from our successes.

The opportunities we see today won't be waiting forever, so we can spend an exorbitant amount of energy trying to calculate every move, or, as with Moses, we can step out boldly in faith fueled by vision to see the possibilities, and prayerfully reflect to adjust our strategy accordingly.

Reflection Questions

1. Have you ever seen God provide you with words to say when you didn't think you had any?

2. Where is God calling you to step out in faith?

CHAPTER 20

WAITING EXPECTANTLY ON GOD

✍

The world I see today is drastically different than the world I used to see before cancer invaded it. I'm still the same person with the same hard wiring, but surprisingly, the long, grueling, and often painful journey of cancer shaped and molded me into a much better version of myself. Moreover, through this journey I discovered that regardless of how much energy I put into a given situation, ultimately my power is limited. No matter what life brings me, I now realize without a shadow of doubt that I can access power beyond myself to get through it. This awesome awareness changed everything for me.

Now when I think about my future, I no longer concern myself with questions that have me wondering what I will do with my life. Instead I ponder thoughts that have me seeking God's will for me. How could it be that this deadly journey sent me on a quest not only to discover who I am but also to understand how God uniquely wired me for his purpose? Daily I'm reminded to pay close attention and wait expectantly on God. I know now that failure to do so may result in a missed opportunity to impact others in a positive way. Seeing my story unfold has been nothing but miraculous. Never in my wildest dreams did I imagine seeing myself as a person whom God has chosen to make a difference in this world. And now that I do, I want to use every breath that remains in me to break down walls, build bridges, and remind others that they too are not alone and have a unique purpose.

Traveling down a difficult road corrected my lens. Before cancer, I saw most people as less than me, but I failed to see the broken state I, too, was in. Now I see myself and everyone on the planet as equals. Instead of putting a lot of effort into making premature judgments, I now disburse my energy differently by paying careful attention to the world around me and seeing the good in others. Amazingly, as I seek to find understanding, I've been more inclined to celebrate the differences in individuals with whom I come in contact. This leaves me dreaming about what could be done with their story.

Although I'm no longer a classroom teacher, my goal remains the same. My desire is to meet people where they are and call out their gifting so that they, too, can take the next step toward influence for good. For everyone, getting started can be intimidating. At first I was unsure about sharing my story, but as I faced my fears, I saw how the experience could be valuable and rewarding. Along the way, it became clear to me that I could give inspiration to others by sharing it too. What gave me courage was knowing that people might notice my exposed vulnerability, and that might give others permission to be vulnerable as well. It is pure joy to see others explore their own stories and find their purpose and passion through them. Come to think of it, there is no greater show on Earth than how God uses willing and passionate individuals as combustible fuel toward creating change.

I learned so many lessons throughout my cancer journey. It has now become very clear to me that sometimes a story doesn't automatically appear after a traumatic incident in one's life—sometimes self-examination can be needed for these stories to emerge. No doubt, this type of reflective thinking will require a person to be introspective, allowing them to go deeper into their thoughts. So, think to yourself, what does the small, still voice inside of you say about your passion? What are you telling yourself you will get to later because you're too busy to find the time for it right now? Or, maybe, what are you holding on to until you finish school, until the kids are out of the house, until you are retired? Remember that tomorrow is not promised.

So, what is *your* story? What passion has God set in your heart?

It is up to you to take the next step of faith, and thankfully it's God's responsibility to provide. God will determine the *how*. All this to say, step out in faith. Life is short. Take a chance. Your story and how you use it will be the greatest gift you can give to this world. After all, it only takes one person to change someone's life.

Not only that, but we also rejoice in our sufferings, knowing that suffering produces endurance, and endurance produces character, and character produces hope, and hope does not put us to shame, because God's love has been poured into our hearts through the Holy Spirit who has been given to us. (Romans 5:3–5)

Reflection Questions

1. What has God uniquely prepared you for or given you a passion for? How can you follow him in that?

2. What one thing will you carry with you after reading this story of God's faithfulness?

DO YOU KNOW SOMEONE
WITH CANCER?

GO TO

PHILSFRIENDS.ORG

to request a care package for
someone you know with cancer,
volunteer and donate.

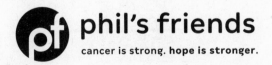

HOW HAVE YOU SEEN
THE GOOD IN IT?

What has God done in your life during a difficult time?

SHARE YOUR STORY BY VIDEO OR EMAIL AT:

SEEINGTHEGOODINIT @PHILSFRIENDS.ORG

Check out other stories at:

PHILSFRIENDS.ORG

or write to us: 213 Wesley Street, Wheaton, IL 60187